Renal Diet Cookbook

An Easy-to-Follow Guide to Cure Kidney Disease with Healthy and Delicious Renal Diet Recipes

© Copyright 2019 - All rights reserved.

The content contained within this book may not be reproduced, duplicated or transmitted without direct written permission from the author or the publisher.

Under no circumstances will any blame or legal responsibility be held against the publisher, or author, for any damages, reparation, or monetary loss due to the information contained within this book. Either directly or indirectly.

Legal Notice:

This book is copyright protected. This book is only for personal use. You cannot amend, distribute, sell, use, quote or paraphrase any part, or the content within this book, without the consent of the author or publisher.

Disclaimer Notice:

Please note the information contained within this document is for educational and entertainment purposes only. All effort has been executed to present accurate, up to date, and reliable, complete information. No warranties of any kind are declared or implied. Readers acknowledge that the author is not engaging in the rendering of legal, financial, medical or professional advice. The content within this book has been derived from various sources. Please consult a licensed professional before attempting any techniques outlined in this book.

By reading this document, the reader agrees that under no circumstances is the author responsible for any losses, direct or indirect, which are incurred as a result of the use of information contained within this document, including, but not limited to, — errors, omissions, or inaccuracies.

Table of Contents

Part I 1

Introduction 2

Chapter 1: Kidney Function 101 4

    New and Exciting Therapies and Treatments for Chronic Kidney Disease 12

Chapter 2: Meal Planning with Kidney Disease . 17

    Kidney Disease Diet for Stages One Though Four 17

    Kidney Disease Diet for Stage Five and Dialysis Patients 22

    Lifestyle Factors 29

Part II 30

Chapter 3: Breakfast 31

    Greek Yogurt Pancakes 31

    Cauliflower Breakfast Hash 34

    Eggs with Green Chilies 37

    Quinoa Breakfast Bowls 40

    Maple Cinnamon French Toast 43

    Single-Serving Blueberry Muffin 46

    Strawberry Scones 49

    Protein-Rich Vegetable Hash 52

Fluffy Belgian Waffles 55

Chapter 4: Snack and Appetizers....................... 58

Roasted Edamame 58

Vanilla Frozen Blueberries 61

Cream Cheese Rangoon Rolls 63

Crispy Chocolate Clusters 66

Creamy Stuffed Celery 68

Tuna Cucumber Bites 70

Peanut Butter Yogurt 72

Parmesan Roasted Cauliflower 74

Crispy Kale Chips 76

Chocolate Strawberry Bites 79

Cinnamon Candied Almonds 82

Chapter 5: Lunch 84

Chicken Fajita Bowls 84

Single Pan Balsamic Chicken and Veggies 87

Pink Salmon with Roasted Broccoli 90

Easy and Gourmet Pasta Salad 93

Greek Chicken Pita Sandwiches 97

Chicken and Rice Soup 100

Barbecue Tofu and Rice 103

Tex-Mex Quinoa Salad 106

Chapter 6: Dinner 109

    Shepherd's Pie.. 109

    Italian Herb Chicken and Asparagus 112

    Baked Chicken Tacos 115

    Mushroom Kale Quesadillas 118

    Creamy Italian Chicken.................................. 121

    Chicken and Rice Scampi 124

    Mushroom Parmesan Pasta............................. 127

    Stuffed Bell Pepper Soup................................ 130

    Seared Chicken and Green Beans.................... 133

    Poached Thai Salmon 136

    The Best Turkey Burgers 139

Chapter 7: Side Dishes..................................... 142

    Lime Cilantro Rice 142

    Spanish Rice.. 145

    Parmesan Quinoa with Peas........................... 147

    Mushroom Orzo 150

    Carrot and Pineapple Slaw 152

    Sesame Cucumber Salad 154

    Creamy Jalapeno Corn.................................. 156

    Crispy Parmesan Cauliflower.......................... 158

    Cucumber Dill Salad with Greek Yogurt Dressing

.... 160

Zesty Green Beans with Almonds 162

Roasted Carrots and Broccoli 164

Tahini and Pomegranate Carrots 166

Chapter 8: Breads 168

Fluffy Sandwich Bread 168

No-Knead Rustic Loaf 171

Pita Bread 174

Italian Focaccia 177

Cinnamon Swirl Loaf 180

French Bread 183

Chapter 9: Desserts 186

Cinnamon Apple Crisp 186

Vanilla Chia Seed Pudding 189

Raspberry Frozen Yogurt 191

Skinny Cheesecake 193

Lemon and Honey Oatmeal Cookies 196

Carrot Cake Cookies 199

Conclusion 202

Part I

Introduction

The kidneys are two bean-shaped organs that we all know about in passing. However, they are still greatly underappreciated. While people may know that they are a set of two organs which are a part of the urinary tract, too few people appreciate and understand the vital importance of these organs. Not only do kidneys help in the production of urine, but they also filter waste and toxins from our blood, remove these particles from our bodies, manage fluid and mineral levels, and synthesize vitamin D so that it can be utilized by our cells. With all of the abilities of our kidneys, people are in a dangerous state when they have chronic kidney disease. Not only does this disease cause a person's kidney disease functioning to lessen, but it also can lead to kidney failure. When a person develops kidney failure, they are unable to survive without either transplantation or blood dialysis treatments multiple times a week.

Sadly, the number of cases of chronic kidney disease is only on the rise in the United States and other Western countries. With high blood pressure and diabetes also on the rise, which is both primary culprits for having kidney disease, the damage to peoples' kidneys is only worsening as time goes on. Without treating both kidney disease and the condition that predisposed a person for the disease, such as high blood pressure or diabetes, a person can not expect to get better.

Thankfully, there is an option. The chronic kidney disease diet does not only treat kidney disease, but it also treats both diabetes and high blood pressure allowing a person to frequently stop the spread of kidney damage. The purpose of this is to hopefully prevent kidney failure before it happens, and if a person does develop kidney failure, to then manage the condition along with other necessary treatments.

In Renal Diet Cookbook, Dr. Robert Porter will help you better understand kidney functioning and health while Dr. Elizabeth Porter provides you with over sixty recipes to enjoy on the kidney disease diet and lifestyle.

No longer do you have to simply accept the progression of chronic kidney disease. You can now use a healthy and delicious renal diet to increase the health of your kidneys and improve your entire life.

Chapter 1: Kidney Function 101

The kidneys are two incredibly powerful organs. When a person has two healthy and fully functioning kidneys, these organs can filter four ounces of blood removing waste and impurities from it every minute. During the process of filtering this blood, not only do the kidneys remove waste, but they also remove a little excess fluid to create urine and remove the waste. After this process, the waste-filled fluid is pushed to the bladder where it will become urine before being expelled from the body.

Since the kidneys filter the blood, people may mistakenly believe that the kidneys are like a sponge that absorbs and hold onto any waste or impurities. However, this is not true. The kidneys may remove waste and toxins from the blood, but rather than holding onto it, they have a process to eliminate it in our system.

The kidneys will also remove some excess acid from your blood, which is a production of your blood used to maintain healthy levels of water and minerals. This acid affects many minerals, but most notably phosphorus, potassium, sodium, and calcium. When these minerals become unbalanced, it leads to a host of problems, such as trouble balancing and an inability of the muscles, tissues, and nerves to function properly. This can become incredibly dangerous.

Since the kidneys cannot manage anymore the levels of acid in your blood or properly manage your mineral levels, it can lead to a dangerous buildup, which is just as damaging to your body as a deficit. For this reason, people with chronic kidney disease (CKD) have to manually manage their mineral intake to prevent buildup.

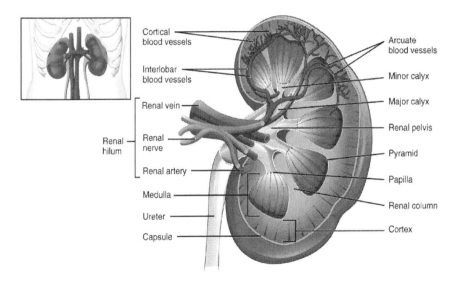

But, who is most at risk of chronic kidney disease? You might be reading this book if you have already been diagnosed, but you may also be reading it if your doctor suspects kidney disease or if a family member has been diagnosed. Therefore, it is important to understand the risk factors of the disease, so that you can better know if you or your loved ones are at risk.

Firstly, people with a family history of kidney disorders, high blood pressure, or diabetes have a higher chance of developing CKD. Although, there are also other people with an increased risk, which include the elderly, black people, Latinx people, Native people, and Pacific Islanders.

There are also many conditions that can directly cause chronic kidney disease. This includes kidney inflammation, high blood pressure, urinary tract infections, renal cancer, and type I and type II diabetes. In fact, renal cancer is one of the most common types of cancer in the United States, being the seventh most common. Two-thirds of the chronic kidney illnesses' cases are because of high blood pressure and diabetes, meaning that not only do people need to treat their kidney health directly, but also indirectly by treating these two conditions. If a person has high blood pressure or diabetes with kidney disease and doesn't treat the former, then these conditions will only worsen kidney health and potentially lead to kidney failure.

If you're at risk of having a disease in your kidneys have increased, your doctor suspects you might have already developed it, then they will likely run a series of tests. These frequently include blood pressure, serum creatinine, and urine albumin tests. If a person experiences increased markers on these three tests, they will likely receive a diagnosis for chronic kidney disease or another kidney condition. Testing for CKD is really simple and a quick process, allowing your doctor to run regular yearly tests if you are concerned about your kidney health due to increased risk of developing the disease.

While chronic kidney disease is one of the more common and dangerous kidney conditions, there are other conditions related to poor kidney health as well. The dangers of CKD is that it can easily cause dangerous side effects if a person doesn't eat well and it can develop into full-on kidney failure.

With chronic kidney disease, when left untreated, a person's kidneys slowly degrade and take on more damage as they decrease in their ability to function. If a person reaches kidney failure, they are in stage five of the disease which is the most severe. With this stage, a person is unable to survive unless they seek medical attention in the way of transplantation or blood dialysis treatment.

If are in need of a transplant down the road, you will be happy to know those healthy individuals can donate their kidneys. Not only can someone donate one of their whole kidneys, but they can also donate simply a portion of their kidneys to help someone who has reached kidney failure. Many people seek to donate their kidneys when a family member or friend is in need, however, it is also possible for people with healthy kidneys to donate their kidneys to strangers in need.

Thankfully, if someone is hoping to donate their kidney, they do not have to worry about its safety. Of course, there are always risks with any surgery no matter how minor. However, kidney removal and transplantation are one of the most common surgeries in the United States, meaning that there is less risk than many other surgeries. If a person is interested in donating an organ, they should contact their doctor who can discuss the risks, benefits, and walk them through the process.

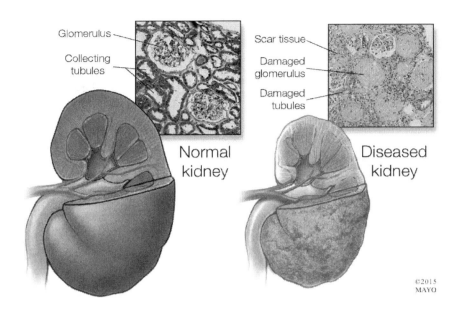

If you are diagnosed with chronic kidney disease, your doctor will use a test known as a glomerular filtration rate (GFR) to understand which stage of the disease you are in. By knowing what stage of the disease you are in, a doctor can better understand how damaged your kidneys are and how likely kidney failure is to develop. Not only that, but your treatment needs and dietary requirements change depending on what level of CKD you are in.

- **Stage One**

    A person has normal GFR results ($\geq$ 90 mL/min/1.73 m2) along with persistent excessive albumin protein in the urine, structural kidney disease, or hereditary kidney disease. Kidney damage may also be viewable through an ultrasound, CT scan, X-ray with contrast, and an MRI.

- **Stage Two**

    GFR results 60 to 89 mL/min/1.73 m2. At this point, the person is unlikely to be experiencing symptoms from the disease. Therefore, if the disease is discovered this early, it is often only due to the treatment of another disease such as diabetes or high blood pressure.

- **Stage Three A.**

    GFR results 45 to 59 mL/min/1.73 m2. A person may start to experience symptoms during stage three (either type A. or B.). These may include fatigue, lower back pain, shortness of breath, swelling, fluid retention, urination changes, muscle cramps, restless legs, or trouble sleeping. These symptoms are the same in both types of stage three.

- **Stage Three B.**

    GFR results 30 to 44 mL/min/1.73 m2

- **Stage Four**

    GFR results 15 to 29 mL/min/1.73 m2. Along with the symptoms in stage three, a person may experience additional symptoms in stage four. These symptoms can include bad breath, taste changes, loss of appetite, vomiting, nausea, difficulty concentrating, and nerve problems such as numbness and tingling.

- **Stage Five**

    GFR results <15 mL/min/1.73 m2. Along with the symptoms of the previous stages, a person in stage five (kidney failure) may experience itching, skin color changes, puffy eyes, and little to no urination.

When you have chronic kidney disease, the most important thing to remember is to always be careful about what you are putting in your body. This, of course, means fluids and foods, but it also includes what medications you take. For instance, many over-the-counter medications are not safe for those with decreased kidney health. Smoking will also decrease your risk.

However, while all lifestyle factors can impact kidney health, in this book, we will be focusing on how diet affects your kidney health and provide you with recipes to maintain a healthy and delicious kidney-friendly diet.

New and Exciting Therapies and Treatments for Chronic Kidney Disease

One common problem of chronic kidney disease is protein leakage from the kidneys. This is known as proteinuria. This problem is dangerous on its own, but it also further worsens kidney disease. Thankfully, there is a brand new and breakthrough drug therapy that can help decrease proteinuria and alleviate some of the damage that it causes. This is a wonderful answer which can decrease future kidney damage in people all around the world.

This new drug therapy uses what is known as a blocker compound, which is combined with another blocker compound frequently in the treatment of high blood pressure and nephropathy in people with type II diabetes. These two blockers are being used in conjunction, as researchers found that they beneficially interact with kidney cell receptors.

Nearly half of the people who have chronic kidney disease also have diabetes, which is startling. Thankfully, there is new hope for patients who have both type II diabetes and chronic kidney disease. In trials on new drug therapy, with the medicine canagliflozin, researchers found that the medication offered new options in reducing the production of the kidney disease. This is especially exciting, as it is the first time in more than fifteen years that success such as this has been reached.

This trial consisted of a large pool of individuals, which means that it is incredibly sound. Four-thousand and four-hundred individuals participated, finding that canagliflozin (sold under Invokana) can help stop the progression of the disease safely. In fact, the trial was able to end sooner than was originally planned, as it was proven to be safe and effective more quickly than researchers had hoped.

While there are some medications that lower blood pressure and reduce the risk of chronic kidney disease, these other medications are only partially effective. On the other hand, Invokana, a small daily pill meant to control blood sugar, has been shown to be much more effective in the reduction in the risk of kidney failure and prevention of chronic kidney disease. The study found that the participants on Invokana experienced a thirty percent lower chances of kidney failure, the requirement for dialysis treatment, required kidney transplantation, or death related to either kidney or heart problems.

Worldwide, there are one hundred and sixty million people with type II diabetes who have a higher chance of having chronic kidney disease. With this new medication option on the horizon, it offers new options in preventing the risk of kidney failure, transplantation, and dialysis. The importance of these results can not be overstated.

In the future, the need for kidney transplantation might decrease. While the demand for transplantation has only increased in recent years, as kidney disease, high blood pressure, and diabetes are on the rise, the future offers new hope. Why is this? It is all thanks to the ongoing research in stem cells and their ability to heal.

While patients won't see the results of stem cell research for years to come, scientists have found several exciting possibilities. For instance, researchers are currently studying how it is possible for the kidneys to regenerate themselves rather than requiring transplantation. To this end, researchers are attempting to discover which type of kidney cells are needed for the process.

As kidney disease is a result of different cell types being damaged in the kidneys, researchers must consider which cells are damaged. This means that stem cell treatments are only effective when researchers know which cells were damaged and need replacement.

While it is still yet to be clear which type of cells are needed for kidney regeneration, there are several groups of cells that are being investigated. Some of these cells that are located around the nephrons possess characteristics similar to stem cells. One of the cell groups currently being investigated is the renal progenitor cells. There is another type of cell that is also being investigated, which is similar to the cells found in bone marrow, known as mesenchymal stem cells.

One type of stem cell being used in ongoing research is the pluripotent stem cells. These cells are being used to create 3D structures similar to the nephrons of our kidneys. The purpose of this is to analyze how they are formed in embryos, test new drug therapy options, and create the possibility of replacing the nephrons on damaged kidneys in the future.

As you can see, there are some exciting new possibilities now available for those with chronic kidney disease, with more opportunities being researched for the future. We discuss more new therapies, treatments, and medications in our other book, *Kidney Disease Diet*.

Chapter 2: Meal Planning with Kidney Disease

In this chapter, we will explore how you can plan your diet while taking the best care of your kidneys as possible. We will look at not only how you should eat when you have chronic kidney disease, but how different stages of the disease can affect your diet.

Kidney Disease Diet for Stages One Though Four

On all stages of the kidney disease diet, you need to limit sodium, potassium, and phosphorus. However, for those who are not on dialysis between stages one and four, protein should also be limited. Overall, your diet should consist of as many fruits and vegetables as you can consume without going over your daily intake of potassium and phosphorus. You want to consume refined grains rather than whole grains, as they are lower in these minerals. The healthier fats, such as olive oil, should be used in place of typically unhealthy fats to improve heart-health and in the process of kidney health.

Nuts, seeds, beans, and lentils can all be enjoyed for their health benefits, but only in moderation due to their high mineral content. And lastly, sugar should be avoided, with only small amounts of natural sweeteners (honey and maple) and in the place of sugar natural alternatives (stevia and sugar alcohols).

Protein is an important aspect of a person's diet as it wards off infections, repairs cellular damage, and prevents muscle wasting. However, protein intake should be closely monitored for a person with chronic kidney disease. For a person in stages one through four, they will most likely be recommended decreased protein consumption by their doctor. While most adults are recommended 0.8 grams of protein per kilogram of body weight, there is not one set recommendation for people with chronic kidney disease. Therefore, you should ask your doctor or renal dietitian about your needed protein daily intake.

For people with chronic kidney disease, it is important to limit protein intake due to the waste byproducts in the protein. For most people, this waste is no problem, as the kidneys can filter it from the body. However, the same is not true of people whose kidneys lack full function. This causes waste to buildup in the bloodstream, worsening kidney damage and increasing the progression of the disease. Thankfully, studies have shown that by limiting protein intake, a person can slow the progression of their disease.

Not all protein is created equal. Try to limit red meat, as this will worsen high blood pressure and heart disease, which is not only bad for your heart, but also for your kidneys. Plant-based proteins are the ideal protein source for chronic kidney disease, as studies have found that by favoring plant-based proteins, people can lessen the progression of their disease. There are multiple reasons for this, partially because animal-based proteins are lower in harmful saturated fats. However, it is also due to the phosphorus found in these foods. Both meat and plant-based proteins contain phosphorus, but it is more bioavailable in meat, meaning that your body absorbs in more. On the other hand, the phosphorus in plant-based proteins has a limited bioavailability, which means less of it is absorbed to affect your kidneys.

Of course, you have to limit many plant-based proteins, such as beans, due to their mineral content. But, when possible, try to consume plant-based proteins such as tofu, edamame, beans, lentils, grains, seeds, and nuts.

There are nine essential amino acids, which are the building blocks of protein. In animal-based products, you get all nine of these needed amino acids. However, many plant-based foods contain only a handful of amino acids. You have to consume a variety of foods to consume all your needed amino acids. Thankfully, there are some sources of complete protein in plant-based products, meaning they have all of these nine amino acids. These complete plant-based proteins are:

- Quinoa
- Buckwheat
- Chia seeds
- Tofu
- Beans paired with rice

While the specific amount of protein a person with chronic kidney disease should eat in a day will vary depending on their doctor's recommendation, a common recommendation is between fifty and sixty grams. Let's look at one way you can consume this amount of protein with a mixture of both plant-based and animal-based proteins:

- Quinoa, cooked - .5 cup

- Yogurt, low-fat - .5 cup
- Beans, cooked - .5 cup
- Chicken breast – 4 ounces

With these few sources of protein throughout your day, you can consume fifty-three grams of protein. These four protein sources, when combined together, also contain 176 milligrams of sodium, 707 milligrams of phosphorus, and 1090 milligrams of potassium.

It is vital for sodium to be limited, which is in much more than just salt. You also find sodium in cheeses, meats, broths, and more. The problem is that these cause high blood pressure and worsen kidney damage. In general, if a person has healthy blood pressure, they can consume between two-thousand and three-thousand milligrams of sodium daily. This means that highly-processed foods, lunch meats, many canned foods (those that are high in sodium), and pre-prepared meals should all be avoided.

Phosphorus easily builds up in the bloodstream, worsening kidney damage. Again, your doctor should recommend a specific daily amount of phosphorus for you in order to limit your intake. The specific amount of phosphorus you can eat will vary, but generally, when a person reaches the end-stage of the disease (stage 5), they are advised to consume no more than one-thousand milligrams daily.

Calcium may be limited, which is not generally difficult, as many foods that are high in calcium are also high in phosphorus, meaning you will already be avoiding them.

Lastly, it is important to limit potassium. While your doctor will recommend a specific daily intake of potassium, in general, people in stages one through four shouldn't consume more than two-thousand milligrams daily. Potassium is a mineral easy to consume, as it is found in high number in many natural and healthy foods. However, when you have kidney disease, your kidneys are no longer able to filter out excess potassium from your bloodstream, causing a dangerous buildup. Therefore, you have to limit it to make up for the inability of your kidneys.

Kidney Disease Diet for Stage Five and Dialysis Patients

The fifth stage of kidney disease, when a person usually begins dialysis unless they receive a transplant, looks different than the diet for stages one through four. In this stage, you need to take more precautions. This generally means you have to watch your mineral intake even more carefully, increase protein intake, and decrease fluid intake. Your doctor will recommend a specific mineral intake based on your needs, so let's look at the fluids and protein in more detail.

Fluids:

Often times, people do not consume enough water. However, people who are undergoing dialysis can easily develop a fluid overload known as hypervolemia. This is dangerous, as it can cause excessive swelling and difficulty in breathing.

When a person experiences kidney failure and begins dialysis, their kidneys are no longer able to balance fluid levels. This can lead to hypervolemia, which is incredibly dangerous. This side effect is the same reason as to why people need to be even more hypervigilant in limiting their sodium intake because sodium will increase the body's fluid levels. Thankfully, by reducing sodium and fluid levels, you can limit this.

If you are worried you might have consumed too much sodium or fluids, watch for telltale symptoms of hypervolemia, such as shortness of breath, cramping, headaches, high blood pressure, bloating, swelling, increased heart rate, and heart palpitations.

The exact amount of fluids you can consume will vary from person to person. Your doctor and dialysis team can discuss with you how many ounces of fluids you can drink in a day, including water, coffee, tea, and broth. However, while there is not one set recommendation, oftentimes, people are recommended no more than thirty-two ounces daily.

Doctors frequently recommend using ice chips, frozen grapes, and sugar-free hard candies to control thirst levels when limiting liquid intake.

Protein:

In general, people are recommended to limit their protein intake in stages one through four of chronic kidney disease. However, when a person is on dialysis in stage five, they are recommended the opposite. Since the process of dialysis can better manage the waste in your bloodstream, patients are instructed to increase healthy sources of protein, as these can help a person increase their overall health.

When increasing your protein, it is important that you don't reach for red meats, as these are high in saturated fats that will worsen blood pressure and kidney damage. Instead, try to enjoy poultry, fish, seafood, eggs, and plant-based proteins. You can also consume certain dairy products, but only in moderation due to their sodium, phosphorus, and potassium contents.

Foods to Enjoy and Avoid for Stages 1-5:

The following is a list of foods that you should avoid and those that you can enjoy. However, it is important to remember that just because something isn't listed here doesn't mean you can't strictly consume it. The foods not listed are often somewhere in-between the avoid and enjoy lists, meaning that you can enjoy them, but only in small quantity. Keep in mind that you can't freely eat as much as you want from the enjoy list, as these foods still contain a certain amount of phosphorus and potassium, meaning you have to take their nutritional data in mind. The easiest way to keep track of what you are eating and ensure you aren't eating too much potassium or phosphorus is to track your food with an app. Many smartphone diet apps will track not only what you eat, but the nutritional data of what you are eating. This means that you can see the number of minerals you are consuming, ensuring you aren't eating too many foods high in these minerals.

Avoid:	Enjoy:
Avocados	Turkey
Dark-colored sodas	Chicken
Whole grains	Salt-free broth/stock
High-sodium canned products	Fish
	Pork
Bananas	Beef
Cantaloupe	Seafood
Honeydew	White bread
Kiwi	White rice
Mango	Couscous
Nectarines	Pasta
Papaya	Pearled barley
Milk (limit dairy in general)	Egg noodles
Processed meats	Almond milk, unsweetened
Oranges	Rice milk, unsweetened
Olives	Soy milk, unsweetened
Pickles	Rice milk, unsweetened
Relish	Apples
Potatoes	Carrots
Sweet Potatoes	Cucumbers

Apricots	Grapes
Tomatoes	Celery
Pre-made meals and highly processed foods	Berries
	Green beans
Dates	Corn
Dried fruits	Radishes
Swiss chard	Peach
Spinach	Cherries
Beet greens	Pineapple
Salty snack foods	Cottage cheese
Seasonings with salt	Parmesan cheese
Chocolate drinks	Feta cheese
Beer	Blue cheese
Regular (non-Greek) yogurt	Greek yogurt
	Cream cheese
Oysters	Neufchatel cheese
Organ meat	Apple juice
Fish roe	Cranberries
Oat bran	Watermelon
Wheat bran	Plums
Brewer's yeast	Pears
Grapefruit juice	Asparagus
Pomegranate juice	Kale
Parsnips	Eggplant
Rutabagas	Cauliflower
Tomatoes	Cabbage

Beets	Onions
Artichoke	Garlic
Squash, both winter and summer	Herbs and spices (free of salt)
Okra	Peppers
Parsnips	Rhubarb
Table salt	Mushrooms
Sea salt	Coffee (limited to 8 ounces
Garlic salt	Tea (limited to 16 ounces)
Seasoning salt	Beans and lentils (in moderation)
Soy sauce	
Onion salt	
Celery salt	
Meat tenderizer	
Lemon pepper.	
Oyster sauce	
Teriyaki sauce	
Barbecue sauce	
Cured foods, such as meats and vegetables	
Lunch meats	

Lifestyle Factors

Keep in mind that it is not only your diet that will affect your kidney health but also your other lifestyle factors. Exercise, sleep quality, alcohol intake, smoking, over the counter medications, and more can affect your kidney health. If you want to treat your chronic kidney disease, you don't only need to begin the kidney disease diet, but take it as a whole life approach, in which you improve various lifestyle factors as well. **How you can improve your lifestyle factors for better kidney health is further discussed in our other book, _Kidney Disease Diet_, also by Dr. Robert Porter and Dr. Elizabeth Torres.**

Part II

Note:

Pictures about medical recipes are Not included within this book.

Dr. Elizabeth Torres used her specialty (dietician specialized in renal diet) to share recipes specifically for the kidney disease diet, complete with easy to follow step-by-step instructions and nutritional information.

You will love these recipes, their ease, how they can benefit your health, and their flavor. These recipes are truly delicious, making the kidney disease diet enjoyable.

Chapter 3: Breakfast

In this chapter, you will find the perfect recipes to start out your morning! You will find low-protein options for stages 1-4 and high-protein options for those in stage 5 on dialysis.

Greek Yogurt Pancakes

These pancakes are quick and easy to whip up, perfect for any day of the week! Try topping them with sugar-free syrup or fresh fruit.

Chronic Kidney Disease Stage: 1-4

The Details:

The Number of Servings: 2

The Time Needed to Prepare: 2 minutes

The Time Required to Cook: 7 minutes

The Total Preparation/Cook Time: 9 minutes

Number of Calories In Individual Servings: 171

Protein Grams: 9

Phosphorus Milligrams: 217

Potassium Milligrams: 240

Sodium Milligrams: 56

Fat Grams: 6

Total Carbohydrates Grams: 19

Net Carbohydrates Grams: 19

The Ingredients:

- Eggs, large – 1
- Greek yogurt, low-fat - .25 cup
- Rice milk – 2 tablespoons
- Baking powder, low-sodium - .5 teaspoon
- All-purpose flour – 1/3 cup
- Olive oil - .5 tablespoon

The Instructions:

1. Combine in a mixing dish the rice milk, Greek yogurt, and egg with a small whisk.
1. Add the all-purpose flour and low-sodium baking powder to the bowl and whisk until everything is well combined. However, try to avoid mixing the pancake mixture too much; it is okay if there are small clumps.

2. Heat an electric griddle or a skillet over medium to medium-high heat. Once hot, grease the skillet with the olive oil and pour the pancake batter into small circles on the pan.

3. Allow the pancakes to cook until the dough is full of air bubbles and begins to look dry, then flip them over. Don't mess with the pancakes unless you are flipping them, as it can cause them to stick or break. Once the other side of the pancakes has become golden, remove them from the skillet and cook any leftover batter.

4. Serve the pancakes immediately with your favorite toppings.

****

Download the Audio Book Version of This Book for FREE.

Copy, and Paste (text precisely) the link into your web browser to get started! https://tinyurl.com/wcobds6 or send an e-mail to: renaldietcookbook@gmail.com

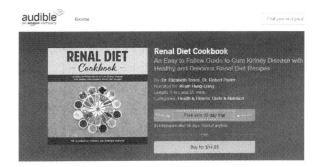

Cauliflower Breakfast Hash

This cauliflower hash makes a wonderful alternative to traditional potato hashes, which are too high in potassium to be allowed on the kidney diet. The spices and herbs will also increase the flavor, making this hash one of your favorites! Don't worry about the fat of the olive oil, as it is a source of heart-healthy fat.

Chronic Kidney Disease Stage: 1-4

The Details:

The Number of Servings: 2

The Time Needed to Prepare: 2 minutes

The Time Required to Cook: 10 minutes

The Total Preparation/Cook Time: 12 minutes

Number of Calories In Individual Servings: 277

Protein Grams: 7

Phosphorus Milligrams: 125

Potassium Milligrams: 304

Sodium Milligrams: 82

Fat Grams: 25

Total Carbohydrates Grams: 7

Net Carbohydrates Grams: 5

The Ingredients:

- Cauliflower florets – 1 cup
- Eggs – 2
- Onion, diced - .25 cup
- Bell pepper, diced - .25 cup
- Paprika – .5 teaspoon
- Cayenne pepper - .25 teaspoon
- Cilantro, dried – 1 teaspoon
- Cumin – .5 teaspoons
- Olive oil – 3 tablespoons

The Instructions:

1. In a small bowl, combine the paprika, cayenne pepper, dried cilantro, and cumin before setting the bowl of spices over to the side for later.
1. Place a large non-stick skillet on the stove over a temperature of medium heat. Add in the olive oil, diced bell pepper, diced onion, and cauliflower

florets. Allow these vegetables to cook together until they become softened, about five minutes.

2. Sprinkle the prepared cumin and paprika spice mixture over the top of the vegetables and stir them together until completely combined. Place a lid over the skillet and continue to sauté the vegetables in the olive oil until the cauliflower is fork-tender. Occasionally remove the lid to stir the vegetables until they are ready.

3. Remove the lid from the skillet and make two "wells" in the vegetables big enough for the eggs. Crack one egg into each of the wells, cover the skillet with the lid again, and allow it to cook until the eggs are set. Remove away from the stove and serve within minutes.

Eggs with Green Chilies

This flavorful egg casserole is the perfect way to get the extra protein needed when on dialysis. Enjoy this for an easy and delicious breakfast or a no-fuss dinner.

Chronic Kidney Disease Stage: 5/Dialysis

The Details:

The Number of Servings: 2

The Time Needed to Prepare: 5 minutes

The Time Required to Cook: 20 minutes

The Total Preparation/Cook Time: 25 minutes

Number of Calories in Individual Servings: 259

Protein Grams: 24

Phosphorus Milligrams: 343

Potassium Milligrams: 384

Sodium Milligrams: 238

Fat Grams: 13

Total Carbohydrates Grams: 8

Net Carbohydrates Grams: 8

The Ingredients:

- Egg whites – 1 cup
- Whole eggs – 1
- Cheddar cheese, shredded, low-sodium – .5 cup
- All-purpose flour – 1 tablespoon
- Black pepper, ground - .125 teaspoon
- Parsley, dried – .5 teaspoon
- Onion, diced - .25 cup
- Garlic, minced – 2 cloves
- Bell pepper, diced - .25 cup
- Green chilled, canned, rinsed – 2 tablespoons

The Instructions:

1. Preheat your oven to a Fahrenheit temperature of three-hundred and fifty degrees and grease a regular-sized loaf pan for the egg casserole.
1. In a medium-sized bowl for the purpose of mixing, whisk together the egg whites and whole egg until the two are completely combined. Whisk in the remaining ingredients.

2. Pour the prepared egg, vegetable, and cheese mixture into the greased loaf pan and then place it in the center of the oven, allowing it to cook until it has set and the eggs are cooked all the way through, about twenty to twenty-five minutes.

Quinoa Breakfast Bowls

These quinoa breakfast bowls are packed with protein and flavor! You will love how the blueberries and cinnamon complement the seeds. This is a wonderful way to start your morning.

Chronic Kidney Disease Stage: 5/Dialysis

The Details:

The Number of Servings: 2

The Time Needed to Prepare: 5 minutes

The Time Required to Cook: 20 minutes

The Total Preparation/Cook Time: 25 minutes

Number of Calories In Individual Servings: 270

Protein Grams: 11

Phosphorus Milligrams: 256

Potassium Milligrams: 376

Sodium Milligrams: 86

Fat Grams: 6

Total Carbohydrates Grams: 44

Net Carbohydrates Grams: 40

The Ingredients:

- Water - .5 cup
- Tofu, silken - .5 cup
- Almond milk - .75 cup
- Quinoa, raw, rinsed well - .5 cup
- Brown sugar – 1.5 tablespoons
- Vanilla extract - .5 teaspoon
- Cinnamon, ground - .25 teaspoon
- Blueberries, fresh - .5 cup

The Instructions:

1. In a blender, combine the silken tofu, water, and almond milk until smooth. This shouldn't take much work, as the tofu is really soft.

1. Once blended, pour the almond milk and tofu mixture in a large casserole and add in the vanilla extract and quinoa. Allow this quinoa mixture to come to a boil over a temperature of medium-high heat. Be sure to stir the mixture occasionally.

2. Once the quinoa boils, lower the heat's intensity and cover it with a lid, allowing it to simmer for fifteen minutes while continuing to stir occasionally.

3. Stir the brown sugar and cinnamon into the quinoa and then allow it to cook with the lid on for an additional five mins or until the quinoa has almost absorbed all of the liquid.

4. Serve the quinoa, topping it with the blueberries.

Maple Cinnamon French Toast

This delicious and simple French toast is a treat that can be enjoyed on all five stages of the kidney disease diet. However, it is important to remember that those in stages 1-4 require a low-protein diet, whereas it is important for those in stage 5 on dialysis to consume a higher protein content. Therefore, those in stage 5 should consider this meal with an added side of protein.

Chronic Kidney Disease Stage: 1-5/Dialysis

The Details:

The Number of Servings: 2

The Time Needed to Prepare: 5 minutes

The Time Required to Cook: 5 minutes

The Total Preparation/Cook Time: 10 minutes

Number of Calories In Individual Servings: 377

Protein Grams: 12

Phosphorus Milligrams: 178

Potassium Milligrams: 175

Sodium Milligrams: 244

Fat Grams: 15

Total Carbohydrates Grams: 43

Net Carbohydrates Grams: 42

The Ingredients:

- Rice milk – 1 cup
- Eggs – 3
- White bread, low-sodium, thickly cut – 4 slices
- Cinnamon - .25 teaspoon
- Olive oil – 1 tablespoon
- Maple syrup – 1 tablespoon
- Vanilla extract - .5 teaspoon

The Instructions:

1. Set a large stewpot over a heat of medium temperature on the stove and add in the olive oil, allowing it to preheat while you quickly assemble the toast. It is best if the skillet is non-stick.
1. In a dish of medium size, crack the eggs and then add in the rice milk, cinnamon, vanilla extract, and maple syrup. Use a whisk to combine a thick liquid, whisking until the egg whites are completely distributed.

2. Once the mixture is done being whisked, add the bread, allowing it to soak for five to fifteen seconds before flipping it over and letting it soak for a few seconds again. The exact amount of time it soaks will depend on the density of the bread you use. You want it to soak long enough that the bread is completely soaked through, but not so long that it begins to fall apart.

3. Add the toast to your skillet and allow the first side to cook until golden brown and it easily is removed from the pan. Don't try to flip it too soon, or else it will stick and fall apart. Once the first side is golden, about two minutes, flip it over and cook the other side for an additional two minutes.

4. Serve the French toast immediately, either plain or with your favorite low-sugar topping.

Single-Serving Blueberry Muffin

This quick and simple single-serving blueberry muffin can be cooked in a mug and the microwave! Of course, if you would like to cook it in the oven, you can do so instead. For cooking this in the oven, simply set an oven or small toaster oven to a Fahrenheit temperature of three-hundred and fifty degrees and allow it to cook until fully set in the center, about twelve minutes.

If you intend to serve this muffin on stage 5/dialysis, you will need it with a side of added protein.

Chronic Kidney Disease Stage: 1-5/Dialysis

The Details:

The Number of Servings: 1

The Time Needed to Prepare: 2 minutes

The Time Required to Cook: 1.5 minutes

The Total Preparation/Cook Time: 3 minutes

Number of Calories In Individual Servings: 245

Protein Grams: 3

Phosphorus Milligrams: 127

Potassium Milligrams: 207

Sodium Milligrams: 25

Fat Grams: 7

Total Carbohydrates Grams: 41

Net Carbohydrates Grams: 40

The Ingredients:

- All-purpose flour - .25 cup
- Baking powder, low-sodium - .25 teaspoon
- Brown sugar – 1 tablespoon
- Olive oil – .5 tablespoons
- Cinnamon – pinch
- Almond milk – 2 tablespoons
- Blueberries – 1 tablespoon

The Instructions:

1. Combine the low-sodium baking powder, brown sugar, all-purpose flour, and cinnamon together in a microwave-safe mug until the baking powder is fully combined into the other ingredients.

1. Add the olive oil and almond milk to the mug and stir the ingredients together, just until incorporated. If needed, you can add an extra

splash of almond milk. Fold in the blueberries, which can be either fresh or frozen.

2. Place your mug of muffin dough in the microwave and allow it to heat on high for ninety seconds. Remove the muffin from the microwave and enjoy it either plain or with a slight drizzle of maple syrup.

Strawberry Scones

These scones are simple to make, but full of flavor and are fluffy! Perfect to enjoy on their own with a dab of butter or with a small amount of your favorite jam.

Chronic Kidney Disease Stage: 1-4

The Details:

The Number of Servings: 2

The Time Needed to Prepare: 5 minutes

The Time Required to Cook: 15 minutes

The Total Preparation/Cook Time: 20 minutes

Number of Calories In Individual Servings: 231

Protein Grams: 4

Phosphorus Milligrams: 127

Potassium Milligrams: 213

Sodium Milligrams: 25

Fat Grams: 10

Total Carbohydrates Grams: 29

Net Carbohydrates Grams: 28

The Ingredients:

- All-purpose flour - .5 cup
- Baking powder, low-sodium - .5 teaspoon
- Olive oil – 1.5 tablespoons
- Egg white – 1 tablespoon
- Almond milk – 2.5 tablespoons
- Sugar – 1 teaspoon
- Strawberries, sliced - .25 cup

The Instructions:

1. Prepare a baking sheet by lining it with kitchen parchment and then set your oven to a Fahrenheit temperature of four-hundred degrees.
1. In a small bowl for the purpose of mixing, combine the all-purpose flour and low-sodium baking powder. Once combined, mix in the olive oil until it forms a crumbly mixture. Add in the egg white, almond milk, and sugar.
2. Once the batter is formed, gently fold the sliced strawberries into the scone mixture.
3. Once the dough is formed, separate it into two portions, and then set these portions onto the

prepared baking sheet. Form each of the two portions into a triangle or circle of even thickness and width. You want the scones to be about one to one and a half inches thick.

4. Place the two prepared scones in the oven and allow them to bake until they just begin to turn slightly golden, and then remove them and allow them to cool for a few minutes. The scones should require about twelve to fifteen minutes in the oven.

Protein-Rich Vegetable Hash

This easy and simple hash is full of vegetables containing half of your daily vegetable needs. When possible, try to use high-quality roasted chicken that is organic and free of antibiotics, as high-quality protein will create less waste in your blood than cheaper protein sources.

Chronic Kidney Disease Stage: 5/Dialysis

The Details:

The Number of Servings: 1

The Time Needed to Prepare: 5 minutes

The Time Required to Cook: 15 minutes

The Total Preparation/Cook Time: 20 minutes

Number of Calories In Individual Servings: 356

Protein Grams: 31

Phosphorus Milligrams: 314

Potassium Milligrams: 439

Sodium Milligrams: 348

Fat Grams: 22

Total Carbohydrates Grams: 5

Net Carbohydrates Grams: 4

The Ingredients:

Radishes, quartered - .5 cup

Mushrooms, sliced - .25 cup

Bell pepper, diced - .25 cup

Chicken breast, roasted – 3 ounces

Feta cheese, crumbled – 1 ounce

Garlic powder - .25 teaspoon

Onion powder -.25 teaspoon

Olive oil – 1 tablespoon

The Instructions:

1. Set your oven to a Fahrenheit temperature of four-hundred and fifty degrees and place the quartered radishes on a baking sheet. Allow these radishes to cook in the oven until they become fork-tender, about fifteen minutes.
1. Once the radishes are done cooking, heat on the stove a large non-stick or cast iron pan with olive oil (one tablespoon) at a temperature of average heat.

2. Add roasted radishes and remaining ingredients into the hot skillet and allow them to cook until deep golden brown. Every few minutes, stir the hash to allow it to cook on all sides, but be careful not to stir it too frequently. You want the hash to be able to sit in the skillet for a minute or two between stirring it, as this will allow the vegetables to sear.

3. Once the hash has reached your preferred level of golden brown, remove it from the skillet and serve it immediately.

Fluffy Belgian Waffles

These Belgian waffles are perfectly fluffy and can be topped with practically anything. Whether you are in the mood for syrup, berries, compote, jam, or even savory toppings, you will find that these waffles are perfection.

If you are on stage five of chronic kidney disease and are on dialysis, keep in mind that these are low in protein and you will need to increase your protein content in your other meals or serve these waffles along with a side of protein.

Chronic Kidney Disease Stage: 1-5/Dialysis

The Details:

The Number of Servings: 1

The Time Needed to Prepare: 5 minutes

The Time Required to Cook: 10 minutes

The Total Preparation/Cook Time: 15 minutes

Number of Calories In Individual Servings: 279

Protein Grams: 6

Phosphorus Milligrams: 172

Potassium Milligrams: 224

Sodium Milligrams: 71

Fat Grams: 13

Total Carbohydrates Grams: 32

Net Carbohydrates Grams: 31

The Ingredients:

- Eggs – 1
- All-purpose flour, .5 cups, plus 1 tablespoon
- Baking powder, low-sodium - .5 teaspoon
- Olive oil – 1.5 tablespoons
- Almond milk - .5 cup
- Sugar - .75 teaspoon

The Instructions:

1. Before you begin to prepare your Belgian waffle batter, begin by preheating your waffle iron. You can use any waffle iron, although a Belgian waffle iron is ideal for fluffy and traditional waffles.

1. Mix in a bowl that is small in size the low-sodium baking powder, all-purpose flour, and sugar. Once combined, create a well in the middle of the mixture and break the egg into it. Combine the mixture lightly with a fork.

2. Add the almond milk and olive oil into the batter, and stir it together until moistened. There may be small clumps, which are okay, but you want to avoid an excessive number of clumps or overly large clumps.

3. Add the waffle batter into the waffle iron being careful to not overfill the iron. Cook the waffle until golden brown, remove it from the waffle iron and then cook the remaining batter.

4. Serve the waffles with your favorite toppings while still fresh and warm.

Chapter 4: Snack and Appetizers

These snacks and appetizers are the perfect way to lift your energy and keep you full all through the afternoon, to increase your appetite before a meal, or to serve at a party with all of your friends. Enjoy these snacks and appetizers whenever you find yourself needing a boost and you are sure to feel better.

Just remember, calculate the phosphorus, potassium, and sodium in these snacks into your daily goal, so that you don't absentmindedly consume too much.

Roasted Edamame

This edamame is the perfect way to lift your energy during the mid-afternoon, as it is a good low to moderate protein snack with heart-healthy olive oil.

Chronic Kidney Disease Stage: 1-5/Dialysis

The Details:

The Number of Servings: 2

The Time Needed to Prepare: 5 minutes

The Time Required to Cook: 15 minutes

The Total Preparation/Cook Time: 20 minutes

Number of Calories In Individual Servings: 279

Protein Grams: 8

Phosphorus Milligrams: 137

Potassium Milligrams: 357

Sodium Milligrams: 6

Fat Grams: 10

Total Carbohydrates Grams: 8

Net Carbohydrates Grams: 4

The Ingredients:

- Edamame, frozen, shelled – 1 cup
- Olive oil – 1 tablespoon
- Black pepper, ground - .25 teaspoon
- Garlic powder - .5 teaspoon
- Onion powder - .5 teaspoon

The Instructions:

1. Preheat your oven by setting it to a Fahrenheit temperature of four-hundred degrees and use a parchment paper in lining a baking sheet.

1. In a bowl, use a towel and dry the edamame until you have gotten all of the liquid off of them. Add in the olive oil and seasonings, tossing the edamame in them until they are completely and evenly coated. Spread the edamame on the prepared pan with kitchen parchment.

2. Place the edamame in the oven and allow it to roast until crispy, about fifteen to eighteen minutes.

Vanilla Frozen Blueberries

These frozen blueberries are coated in yogurt and lemon juice, giving them a sweet, creamy, and tangy taste. Perfect for a warm summer day, you will absolutely love these blueberries!

Chronic Kidney Disease Stage: 1-5/Dialysis

The Details:

The Number of Servings: 2

The Time Needed to Prepare: 10 minutes

The Time Required to Freeze: 2 hours

The Total Preparation/Cook Time: 130 minutes

Number of Calories In Individual Servings: 91

Protein Grams: 3

Phosphorus Milligrams: 86

Potassium Milligrams: 184

Sodium Milligrams: 38

Fat Grams: 1

Total Carbohydrates Grams: 18

Net Carbohydrates Grams: 17

The Ingredients:

- Blueberries – 1 cup
- Lemon juice – 1 teaspoon
- Vanilla yogurt, low-fat – 4 ounces

The Instructions:

1. Ensure that your blueberries are washed and dry, and then toss them in a bowl along with the lemon juice and yogurt. While doing this, be very gentle as you don't want the blueberries to become squished.

1. One by one, use a spoon or your hands to scoop out each blueberry, setting it on a baking sheet lined with kitchen parchment or wax paper. Ensure that the blueberries are not touching each other on the pan.

2. Place the baking sheet in the freezer and allow them to freeze for two hours. Remove the blueberries from the pan, setting them in either a plastic bag or container and store them in the freezer until you are ready to enjoy.

Cream Cheese Rangoon Rolls

These cream cheese rangoons are the perfect appetizer for any party. However, they are also so easy and quick to make that you can enjoy them any day of the week. Enjoy these alone or paired with your favorite low-sodium dipping sauce.

Chronic Kidney Disease Stage: 1-5/Dialysis

The Details:

The Number of Servings: 2

The Time Needed to Prepare: 5 minutes

The Time Required to Cook: 15 minutes

The Total Preparation/Cook Time: 20 minutes

Number of Calories In Individual Servings: 324

Protein Grams: 8

Phosphorus Milligrams: 83

Potassium Milligrams: 99

Sodium Milligrams: 470

Fat Grams: 15

Total Carbohydrates Grams: 38

Net Carbohydrates Grams: 37

The Ingredients:

- Egg roll wrappers – 4
- Cream cheese, softened – 2 ounces
- Garlic powder - .125 teaspoon
- Olive oil – 2 teaspoons
- Green onions, finely chopped – 1 tablespoon

The Instructions:

1. Prepare a baking sheet by coating it in kitchen parchment and preheat your oven to a Fahrenheit temperature of three-hundred and seventy-five degrees.

1. In a small-scaled dish, put together the green onions with the garlic powder and softened cream cheese.

2. In a small dish, add a small amount of water that you can dip your fingers in, and in another small dish, add your olive oil.

3. Lay out the four egg roll wrappers and divide the prepared cream cheese mixture between them. Place the cream cheese mixture on the bottom edge of the egg roll wrapper, keeping in mind it

will expand as it cooks, so it's okay if it doesn't reach all the edges.

4. Dip your fingers in the prepared dish of water and then run your fingers along the top of the egg roll wrap, on the opposite side from the cream cheese. Ensure that you generously moisten the wrap.

5. Tightly wrap the egg roll wrap around the cream cheese, allowing the water to tightly seal it shut. If needed, you can add more water.

6. After the egg rolls are all tightly wrapped, place them on the prepared baking sheet and allow them to cook for twelve to fifteen minutes until they are golden brown. You should flip them over halfway through the cooking process to ensure they cook evenly.

7. Serve the rolls alone or serve them alongside a kidney diet-friendly sauce that is low in sodium, phosphorus, and potassium.

Crispy Chocolate Clusters

No longer do you have to wish for sugar-laden chocolate bars. Instead, you can enjoy these homemade crispy rice and chocolate clusters. These use coconut oil, which is higher in saturated fat than olive oil, although it is a healthier type of saturated fat than what is found in animal-based products. In fact, coconut oil has been found to have many heart-healthy benefits. You can not replace the coconut oil with another, as coconut oil sets up firm when chilled, whereas many other oils do not.

Chronic Kidney Disease Stage: 1-5/Dialysis

The Details:

The Number of Servings: 2

The Time Needed to Prepare: 5 minutes

The Time Required to Cook: 15 minutes

The Total Preparation/Cook Time: 20 minutes

Number of Calories In Individual Servings: 114

Protein Grams: 8

Phosphorus Milligrams: 13

Potassium Milligrams: 64

Sodium Milligrams: 1

Fat Grams: 9

Total Carbohydrates Grams: 8

Net Carbohydrates Grams: 8

The Ingredients:

- Puffed white rice, plain - .25 cup
- Cocoa – 2 teaspoons
- Vanilla extract – .125 teaspoon
- Maple syrup – 2 teaspoons
- Coconut oil, melted – 4 teaspoons

The Instructions:

1. Together, in a small kitchen bowl, whisk the cocoa powder, vanilla extract, maple syrup, and melted coconut oil. Once it is completely smooth without any clumps, fold in the puffed white rice.
1. Use either a wax or parchment paper in lining a baking sheet. Then, use a spoon and create four mounds of the chocolate rice mixture on the baking sheet.
2. Place the baking sheet in the freezer for an hour until the mounds are flat. Remove them from the baking sheet and then store them either in a plastic bag or container until you are ready to enjoy.

Creamy Stuffed Celery

These celery boats are a much more fun and delicious version than your childhood snack of peanut butter and celery. You will love how the cream cheese and cheddar perfectly accent the celery.

Keep in mind that this recipe uses garlic powder, which is different from garlic salt. Don't ever use garlic salt on the kidney disease diet, as it is high in sodium.

Chronic Kidney Disease Stage: 1-5/Dialysis

The Details:

The Number of Servings: 2

The Time Needed to Prepare: 5 minutes

The Time Required to Cook: 0 minutes

The Total Preparation/Cook Time: 5 minutes

Number of Calories In Individual Servings: 255

Protein Grams: 6

Phosphorus Milligrams: 177

Potassium Milligrams: 219

Sodium Milligrams: 241

Fat Grams: 23

Total Carbohydrates Grams: 4

Net Carbohydrates Grams: 4

The Ingredients:

- Celery stalks, washed and dried – 2
- Cream cheese, softened – 4 ounces
- Cheddar cheese, low-sodium, grated - .25 cup
- Parsley, fresh, chopped – 2 teaspoons
- Chives, chopped – 2 teaspoons
- Black pepper, ground - .125 teaspoon
- Garlic powder - .125 teaspoon

The Instructions:

1. Slice your celery sticks into thirds or quarters, and then set them aside.
1. In a small bowl for the purpose of mixing, add the cream cheese, cheddar cheese, parsley, chives, black pepper, and garlic powder. Using a hand-held kitchen beater, whip the cream cheese mixture so that it is smooth and creamy.
2. Using a small spoon, fill the celery sticks with the cream cheese mixture and then serve immediately or store in the fridge and enjoy later in the afternoon.

Tuna Cucumber Bites

These tuna bites are the perfect way to increase your protein intake. Not only that, but they are delicious and easy to make!

Chronic Kidney Disease Stage: 5/Dialysis

The Details:

The Number of Servings: 2

The Time Needed to Prepare: 5 minutes

The Time Required to Cook: 0 minutes

The Total Preparation/Cook Time: 5 minutes

Number of Calories In Individual Servings: 118

Protein Grams: 19

Phosphorus Milligrams: 181

Potassium Milligrams: 370

Sodium Milligrams: 210

Fat Grams: 2

Total Carbohydrates Grams: 5

Net Carbohydrates Grams: 4

The Ingredients:

Tuna, light, canned – 1 can

Tofu, soft - .33 cup

Onion, thinly sliced - .33 cup

Cucumber, sliced – 1

Black pepper, ground - .25 teaspoon

Garlic powder - .25 teaspoon

The Instructions:

1. Place the black pepper, powder, and soft tofu garlic together in a bowl and then mash them together with a fork until the tofu is broken down.

1. Drain the light tuna and then add it to the tofu mixture along with the thinly sliced onion, and stir the mixture together until it is fully combined.

2. Slice your cucumber and then place the slices on a plate and top the slices off with the tuna mixture. Serve the tuna slices immediately.

Peanut Butter Yogurt

Enjoy this creamy and delicious yogurt either on its own or with a kidney disease diet-friendly fruit or cracker. Celery is even a good option!

Chronic Kidney Disease Stage: 5/Dialysis

The Details:

The Number of Servings: 2

The Time Needed to Prepare: 5 minutes

The Time Required to Cook: 0 minutes

The Total Preparation/Cook Time: 5 minutes

Number of Calories In Individual Servings: 264

Protein Grams: 15

Phosphorus Milligrams: 199

Potassium Milligrams: 346

Sodium Milligrams: 31

Fat Grams: 16

Total Carbohydrates Grams: 18

Net Carbohydrates Grams: 16

The Ingredients:

- Plain Greek yogurt - .5 cup
- Creamy peanut butter, low-sodium/no salt - .25 cup
- Honey – 1 tablespoon

The Instructions:

1. Using a whisk, combine together the plain Greek yogurt, creamy peanut butter, and honey until it is smooth and without clumps. Serve it immediately or save it in the fridge to enjoy at a later date.

Parmesan Roasted Cauliflower

This roasted cauliflower is simple but absolutely delicious! Enjoy it served alone, or you can dip it in a low-sodium homemade mayonnaise made with olive oil.

Chronic Kidney Disease Stage: 1-5/Dialysis

The Details:

The Number of Servings: 2

The Time Needed to Prepare: 5 minutes

The Time Required to Cook: 20 minutes

The Total Preparation/Cook Time: 25 minutes

Number of Calories In Individual Servings: 144

Protein Grams: 5

Phosphorus Milligrams: 131

Potassium Milligrams: 360

Sodium Milligrams: 259

Fat Grams: 10

Total Carbohydrates Grams: 8

Net Carbohydrates Grams: 6

The Ingredients:

- Cauliflower florets – 2 cups
- Olive oil – 1 tablespoon
- Garlic powder - .5 teaspoon
- Black pepper, ground - .125 teaspoon
- Onion powder - .5 teaspoon
- Parmesan cheese, grated - .25 cup

The Instructions:

1. Preheat your oven to a temperature of four-hundred degrees Fahrenheit and then coat a cooking sheet with kitchen parchment.
1. In a mixing pot, blend together the grated Parmesan, onion powder, black pepper, garlic powder, olive oil, and cauliflower florets. Once the cauliflower is fully coated, transfer it to the prepared baking sheet.
2. Roast the cauliflower until golden brown and tender (20 mins). Remove the sheet from the oven and enjoy it immediately while still warm.

Crispy Kale Chips

These kale chips are quick and easy to cook, and they are incredibly healthy! If you want a small snack, but don't want to add to many added minerals or protein to your daily diet, then you can easily enjoy these and only increase your mineral content by a small amount. These are the perfect snack to enjoy when you are watching a movie and want a savory treat in place of popcorn.

Chronic Kidney Disease Stage: 1-5/Dialysis

The Details:

The Number of Servings: 2

The Time Needed to Prepare: 5 minutes

The Time Required to Cook: 20 minutes

The Total Preparation/Cook Time: 25 minutes

Number of Calories In Individual Servings: 130

Protein Grams: 0

Phosphorus Milligrams: 19

Potassium Milligrams: 97

Sodium Milligrams: 8

Fat Grams: 13

Total Carbohydrates Grams: 2

Net Carbohydrates Grams: 2

The Ingredients:

- Kale, chopped – 2 cups
- Olive oil – 2 tablespoons
- Onion powder - -25 teaspoon
- Onion powder - .25 teaspoon
- Parsley, dried - .5 teaspoon
- Dill weed, dried - .5 teaspoon
- Chives, dried - .5 teaspoon

The Instructions:

1. Preheat your oven to a Fahrenheit temperature of two-hundred and seventy-five degrees and then use a kitchen parchment when lining a baking pan.

1. Wash the kale leaves, ensure that they are dried completely, and then cut them into bite-sized pieces. Keep in mind that the leaves will shrink a small amount while they cook.

2. Place the kale in a large kitchen casserole and then blend them with the olive oil and seasoning until they are fully and evenly coated.

3. Lay the seasoned kale leaves out on the prepared cooking sheet in a single layer so that they do not overlap. This is important, as it ensures that the leaves cook evenly and become crispy.

4. Allow the kale to cook for ten minutes before flipping the leaves over and cooking an additional ten minutes until golden and crispy.

5. Serve the kale leaves immediately while hot, or let them cool and then store them in a plastic container to enjoy later on.

Chocolate Strawberry Bites

One of the great things about these strawberry bites is that you don't have to sit down and eat a full serving. While you can certainly enjoy a full serving if you only want one or two bites of sweetness, that's all you have to grab out of the freezer, as they can be stored ready and waiting for you to enjoy. Whether you have just gotten off of work or finished cleaning the kitchen, you can easily enjoy just one or two of these bites for a sweet treat without adding too many extra minerals to your daily diet.

Chronic Kidney Disease Stage: 1-5/Dialysis

The Details:

The Number of Servings: 2

The Time Needed to Prepare: 10 minutes

The Time Required to Freeze: 60 minutes

The Total Preparation/Cook Time: 70 minutes

Number of Calories In Individual Servings: 396

Protein Grams: 4

Phosphorus Milligrams: 188

Potassium Milligrams: 492

Sodium Milligrams: 12

Fat Grams: 28

Total Carbohydrates Grams: 30

Net Carbohydrates Grams: 23

The Ingredients:

- Strawberries, fresh - .25 pound
- Dark chocolate chips – 4 ounces
- Coconut oil – 2 teaspoons

The Instructions:

1. Slice the strawberries into quarters if they are large or in half if they are small. You want them in small bite-size pieces. Get a baking sheet ready with a wax or parchment paper.//
1. In a microwave-safe bowl, add the dark chocolate chips and coconut oil, and then melt them in the microwave. In order to do this, microwave the chocolate for thirty seconds at a time, stirring it at the end of each thirty seconds until the chocolate is fully melted. Don't microwave them for longer periods without stirring, or else, the chocolate might burn.

2. Using a toothpick, pick up each strawberry piece and dip it in the chocolate mixture allowing it to become fully coated. Place the strawberry pieces on the prepared baking sheet when they are coated in chocolate

3. Place the strawberries in the freezer and allow them to chill until fully frozen, at least an hour. Once the chocolate is hardened, remove the frozen strawberries from the pan and put them in a container to be stored in the freezer until serving.

Cinnamon Candied Almonds

These almonds are full of flavor and much healthier than their sugary alternative! These use Truvia sweetener, which is a combination of sugar alcohol and stevia herb, which has been found safe in patients with kidney disease. The benefit of this is that unlike sugar, these will not worsen high blood sugar. Almonds are also a wonderful source of healthy fats and fiber, making them a known superfood.

Chronic Kidney Disease Stage: 1-5/Dialysis

The Details:

The Number of Servings: 2

The Time Needed to Prepare: 2 minutes

The Time Required to Cook: 7 minutes

The Total Preparation/Cook Time: 9 minutes

Number of Calories In Individual Servings: 212

Protein Grams: 7

Phosphorus Milligrams: 173

Potassium Milligrams: 268

Sodium Milligrams: 1

Fat Grams: 17

Total Carbohydrates Grams: 8

Net Carbohydrates Grams: 3

The Ingredients:

- Truvia sweetener – .25 cup
- Almonds, raw – .5 cup
- Cinnamon – 1 teaspoon
- Water – 1 tablespoon
- Vanilla extract - .25 teaspoon

The Instructions:

1. Place a skillet over medium heat and allow it to warm up. Once the skillet is hot, add in the Truvia sweetener, water, cinnamon, and vanilla extract. Using a spoon, combine the mixture and continue to stir it while it melts.

1. Once the Truvia mixture has completely melted, add in the almonds and stir to coat the almonds completely. Continue to stir and cook until the mixture begins to crystallize to the almonds, and then remove it from the heat.

2. Allow the almonds to sit for two to three minutes, and then use a spatula to break them apart before they stick together.

3. Allow the almonds to cool before serving them.

Chapter 5: Lunch

These lunches are perfect complete meals to enjoy in the afternoon, whether you are at home, the office, or on the road. You will be happy to know that these dishes are incredibly simple and easy to cook and are balanced meals.

Chicken Fajita Bowls

This meal is a perfect balance of meat, vegetables, and grains making it a great option to enjoy for lunch or dinner. You can easily serve this meal immediately or make it ahead of time and save it in the fridge to take with you to work for lunch.

Chronic Kidney Disease Stage: 1-4

The Details:

The Number of Servings: 2

The Time Needed to Prepare: 5 minutes

The Time Required to Cook: 15 minutes

The Total Preparation/Cook Time: 20 minutes

Number of Calories In Individual Servings: 365

Protein Grams: 17

Phosphorus Milligrams: 229

Potassium Milligrams: 510

Sodium Milligrams: 46

Fat Grams: 11

Total Carbohydrates Grams: 47

Net Carbohydrates Grams: 45

The Ingredients:

- Chicken breast - .25 pound
- Olive oil – 1.5 tablespoons
- Onion – 1
- Bell pepper, green – 1
- Bell pepper, red – 1
- Garlic, minced – 4 cloves
- Chili powder - .25 teaspoon
- Cayenne pepper – pinch
- Paprika - .25 teaspoon
- Cumin - .25 teaspoon
- Black pepper, ground - .25 teaspoon

- White rice, cooked – 1.5 cups

The Instructions:

1. Combine the chili powder, cayenne pepper, paprika, cumin, and black pepper together to make your fajita seasonings and then set the spices aside.

1. Slice the chicken breast into bite-sized cubes and then place it in a small bowl, massaging it with half of the prepared seasoning mix. Allow it to marinate for fifteen minutes.

2. In a large-sized cooking pan warmed in a stove heat of medium with one tbps of the olive oil, cook the bell pepper and onion until soft, about five mins.

3. Add in the chicken and garlic, and continue to cook until the chicken is fully cooked through, reaching an internal Fahrenheit temperature of one-hundred and sixty-five degrees. This should take about ten minutes. Don't forget to stir the chicken occasionally.

4. The skillet should then be removed away from the stove's heat. Serve the vegetables and chicken over the rice.

Single Pan Balsamic Chicken and Veggies

This chicken and vegetable recipe is incredibly simple and only requires one pan! You can enjoy it either immediately for a fresh dinner or save it in the fridge or freezer for an easy lunch during the week.

Chronic Kidney Disease Stage: 1-4

The Details:

The Number of Servings: 2

The Time Needed to Prepare: 5 minutes

The Time Required to Cook: 15 minutes

The Total Preparation/Cook Time: 20 minutes

Number of Calories In Individual Servings: 346

Protein Grams: 18

Phosphorus Milligrams: 208

Potassium Milligrams: 504

Sodium Milligrams: 89

Fat Grams: 8

Total Carbohydrates Grams: 48

Net Carbohydrates Grams: 45

The Ingredients:

- Chicken, breast, cut into bite-sized pieces - .33 pound
- Baby carrots – 1 cup
- Onion, sliced – 1
- Italian herb seasoning – 1 teaspoon
- Balsamic vinegar – 1 tablespoon
- Olive oil – 1 tablespoon
- Black pepper, ground - .25 teaspoon
- Garlic, minced – 4 cloves
- Rice, white, cooked – 1.5 cups

The Instructions:

1. Preheat your oven to a Fahrenheit temperature of four-hundred degrees before lining a parchment paper in the tray for baking.
1. In a small bowl, use a whisk to combine together the olive oil, balsamic vinegar, Italian herb seasoning, black pepper, and minced garlic.
2. Place the bite-sized chicken pieces in a bowl and add in half of the vinegar and seasoning mix, massaging the mixture into the chicken. Allow the

chicken to marinate for fifteen to thirty minutes ideally or use it right away.

3. Place the chicken and vegetables on the pan and toss them in the remaining prepared seasoning and vinegar mixture until evenly coated. Spread the vegetables and chicken out on the pan so that they cook evenly, and then set the pan into the center of your preheated oven.

4. Cook the mixture for fifteen minutes before turning the pan around to allow for even cooking, and then continue to cook for an additional fifteen minutes. Check and make sure that the chicken has reached an internal Fahrenheit temperature of one-hundred and sixty-five degrees. Remove the pan from the oven if it is ready, and if not, allow it to cook for a few more minutes.

5. Serve the vegetables and chicken over rice, either immediately or save them for lunch later in the week.

Pink Salmon with Roasted Broccoli

This salmon and roasted broccoli are delicious and extremely easy! Just keep in mind that the salmon is higher in potassium than poultry. However, as long as you make sure that the meals you eat during the remainder of your day don't put you over your potassium goal, then you should be okay. It is a good thing to include healthy fatty fish, such as salmon, which you can, as it has many health benefits and vital omega-3 fatty acids.

Chronic Kidney Disease Stage: 1-4

The Details:

The Number of Servings: 2

The Time Needed to Prepare: 5 minutes

The Time Required to Cook: 15 minutes

The Total Preparation/Cook Time: 20 minutes

Number of Calories In Individual Servings: 318

Protein Grams: 21

Phosphorus Milligrams: 301

Potassium Milligrams: 515

Sodium Milligrams: 81

Fat Grams: 11

Total Carbohydrates Grams: 32

Net Carbohydrates Grams: 31

The Ingredients:

- Salmon fillets – 6 ounces
- Cumin - .25 teaspoon
- Broccoli florets – 1 cup
- Olive oil – 1 tablespoon
- Lemon zest - .25 teaspoon
- Lemon juice – 2 teaspoons
- Garlic, minced – 2 cloves
- Red pepper flakes - .125 teaspoon
- Thyme, dried - .25 teaspoon
- Rice, white, cooked – 1.25 cups

The Instructions:

1. Preheat your oven to a Fahrenheit temperature of four-hundred and twenty-five degrees and line a baking pan with kitchen parchment.
1. In a baking sheet, lay down the broccoli florets, add the olive oil over the top, and toss the florets

in the oil until they are evenly coated. Spread the florets around the pan.

2. Set the salmon fillets on the baking pan between the broccoli florets.

3. In a small bowl, combine the lemon zest, cumin, lemon juice, garlic, red pepper flakes, and thyme. Spread this mixture over the top of the salmon. Set the pan in the oven and allow it to cook until the salmon is cooked through and flaky, about ten to fifteen minutes.

4. Withdraw from the oven the baking sheet and serve the rice, vegetables, and fish together. You may want to give a squeeze of fresh lemon over the top of it. It is also nice to add a little extra dried thyme and black pepper to the cooked rice.

Easy and Gourmet Pasta Salad

This pasta salad is full of nutrition, with homemade turkey meatballs, fresh mushrooms and asparagus, and heart-healthy olive oil. Enjoy this dish either immediately after making it, or enjoy it later on as a cold refrigerated treat.

Chronic Kidney Disease Stage: 1-4

The Details:

The Number of Servings: 2

The Time Needed to Prepare: 5 minutes

The Time Required to Cook: 20 minutes

The Total Preparation/Cook Time: 25 minutes

Number of Calories In Individual Servings: 474

Protein Grams: 22

Phosphorus Milligrams: 257

Potassium Milligrams: 419

Sodium Milligrams: 65

Fat Grams: 11

Total Carbohydrates Grams: 52

Net Carbohydrates Grams: 48

The Ingredients:

- Pasta, cooked – 2 cups
- Turkey, ground - .25 pound
- Italian seasoning – 1 teaspoon
- Bread crumbs, plain without seasonings – 1 tablespoon
- Black pepper, ground - .25 teaspoon
- Garlic minced – 3 cloves
- Mushrooms, sliced – .5 cup
- Asparagus - .25 pound
- Olive oil – 2 tablespoons
- Balsamic vinegar – 1 tablespoon

The Instructions:

1. Start boiling a pot of water and let the pasta cook as per instructions. Meanwhile, preheat a saucepan of large size over a stove's medium heat temperature. Preferably, you want to use a non-stick skillet.
1. While the skillet preheats, combine the ground turkey with the breadcrumbs, black pepper, minced garlic, and half of the Italian seasoning. Be

careful not to over mix the meat, otherwise, it will become tough.

2. Using a spoon, scoop out easily-sized portions and then roll them between your hands to form balls. You want each meatball to contain about two to three teaspoons of meat. Just be sure you don't heap the meat over the edge of the tablespoon, or else you will have too much meat mixture.

3. Add one tablespoon of the olive oil to the skillet, add in the rolled meatballs, and cook the meatballs until cooked all the way through with no pink in the center. The middle needs to reach a Fahrenheit temperature of one-hundred and sixty-five degrees Fahrenheit. Be sure to stir the meatballs around occasionally so that all sides can cook!

4. Once the meatballs are done cooking, remove and put them to the side for a while. Add the mushrooms and asparagus to the cooking pot, allowing them to cook until tender, about seven to nine minutes. Remove the skillet from the heat.

5. In a medium-sized bowl, add the cooked pasta, meatballs, and vegetables along with the remaining Italian seasoning, one tablespoon of

olive oil, and the balsamic vinegar. Toss all of the ingredients together and serve it warm, or chill it in the fridge before serving.

Greek Chicken Pita Sandwiches

For these pita sandwiches, be sure that you don't use whole-wheat or enriched pita bread, you want to use white pita bread as it is lowest in phosphorus and potassium. When making this recipe, please keep in mind that while this recipe uses onion and garlic powder, these are not the same as garlic and onion salt. These are different ingredients, as the powder contains much less sodium than the salt variety.

Chronic Kidney Disease Stage: 1-4

The Details:

The Number of Servings: 2

The Time Needed to Prepare: 5 minutes

The Time Required to Cook: 25 minutes

The Total Preparation/Cook Time: 30 minutes

Number of Calories In Individual Servings: 152

Protein Grams: 15

Phosphorus Milligrams: 257

Potassium Milligrams: 419

Sodium Milligrams: 65

Fat Grams: 5

Total Carbohydrates Grams: 9

Net Carbohydrates Grams: 7

The Ingredients:

- Chicken breast, cut into strips - .25 pound
- Onion powder - .25 teaspoon
- Black pepper, ground - .25 teaspoon
- Dill, dried - .5 teaspoon
- Parsley, dried – 1 teaspoon
- Garlic powder - .25 teaspoon
- Sesame seed oil - .5 teaspoon
- Cucumber, thinly sliced – 1
- Lettuce – 1 cup
- Pita bread – 2
- Hummus - .25 cup

The Instructions:

1. Preheat your oven to a Fahrenheit temperature of four-hundred degrees.

2. Place the chicken strips on a small baking sheet and toss them together with the onion powder, black pepper, dried dill, dried parsley, garlic powder, and sesame seed oil. Ensure that they are fully coated and then place it in the oven until the chicken strips are fully cooked. This should take twenty to twenty-five minutes. The middle of the chicken must reach a minimum Fahrenheit temperature of one-hundred and sixty-five degrees.

3. Once the chicken is done cooking, remove it from the oven and prepare the remaining aspects of your sandwiches. You need to cut the pita breads in half and then open the pockets with your hands or a fork. Slice the cucumbers and tear the lettuce into bite-sized pieces.

4. First, fill the pita bread halves with the lettuce, then the cucumber, and lastly, the cooked chicken strips. Serve it immediately to prevent the pita from going stale and while the chicken is still warm.

Chicken and Rice Soup

This soup is quick and easy to make and perfect for a cold winter day or for whenever you are feeling under the weather. However, keep in mind that you should plan this soup for on a day that you have other low-potassium meals planned. This is because while this soup is still classified as low-potassium, it does contain a little more potassium than many of the other recipes in this book.

While you can use low-sodium chicken broth from the store, you are best off using completely homemade broth so that you can ensure it has no added sodium.

Chronic Kidney Disease Stage: 1-4

The Details:

The Number of Servings: 2

The Time Needed to Prepare: 5 minutes

The Time Required to Cook: 25 minutes

The Total Preparation/Cook Time: 25 minutes

Number of Calories In Individual Servings: 374

Protein Grams: 19

Phosphorus Milligrams: 248

Potassium Milligrams: 649

Sodium Milligrams: 122

Fat Grams: 9

Total Carbohydrates Grams: 51

Net Carbohydrates Grams: 48

The Ingredients:

- Water – 2 cups
- Chicken broth, low-sodium – 1 cup
- Onion, dehydrated flakes – 1 tablespoon
- Garlic, minced – 4 cloves
- Celery, diced – 1 rib
- Carrots, sliced – 2
- Chicken breast, sliced into small cubes - .25 pound
- White rice, raw - .5 cup
- Poultry seasoning - .5 teaspoon
- Black pepper, ground - .25 teaspoon
- Olive oil – 1 tablespoon

The Instructions:

1. Place the carrots, celery, garlic, and olive oil in a big casserole. Cook them over medium heat. Allow

these to sauté together for five minutes and then add in the remaining ingredients. Stir the pot together well and bring it to a boil over medium-high heat.

1. Once the pot comes to a boil, reduce it to a simmer, cover it with a lid, and allow it to cook until the rice and chicken are cooked about twenty minutes.
2. Turn off the heat, allow the soup to sit for five minutes, and then serve.

Barbecue Tofu and Rice

This recipe makes faux-barbecue tofu. While barbecue sauce is not allowed on the kidney disease diet due to its high sodium and potassium contents, this recipe utilizes seasonings to make a similar barbecue flavor, but without the use of sodium or potassium-rich tomatoes. If you are a barbecue lover, you will absolutely love this tofu! Of course, you can also make it with chicken, if you wish.

This recipe makes use of onion powder and garlic powder; please keep in mind that these are very different from onion and garlic salt. Unlike the latter, these do not contain added sodium and can be used on the diet for kidney disease.

Chronic Kidney Disease Stage: 5/Dialysis

The Details:

The Number of Servings: 2

The Time Needed to Prepare: 5 minutes

The Time Required to Cook: 15 minutes

The Total Preparation/Cook Time: 20 minutes

Number of Calories In Individual Servings: 462

Protein Grams: 25

Phosphorus Milligrams: 368

Potassium Milligrams: 393

Sodium Milligrams: 23

Fat Grams: 20

Total Carbohydrates Grams: 46

Net Carbohydrates Grams: 44

The Ingredients:

- Tofu, extra firm, cut into bite-sized cubes – 16 ounces
- Corn starch – 1 tablespoon
- Red wine vinegar – 2 tablespoons
- Onion powder - .25 teaspoon
- Cayenne pepper - .125 teaspoon
- Smoked paprika - 1 teaspoon
- Brown sugar – 2 teaspoons
- Olive oil – 2 tablespoons
- Garlic powder - .25 teaspoon
- Black pepper, ground - .25 teaspoon

- Rice, white, cooked - .1.5 cups

The Instructions:

- Add the olive oil in a pan that is warmed over a heat of medium height. While you can use a stainless steel skillet, it is easier to use a non-stick skillet.

- In a medium-sized bowl, add in the corn starch, cayenne pepper, onion powder, smoked paprika, garlic powder, black ground pepper, and brown sugar. Whisk these together and then add in the tofu, tossing them together until the tofu is fully coated. Add in the red wine vinegar and toss the mixture together again.

- Place the tofu cubes in the hot oil of the skillet, giving them each a little space between the cubes so that they are not sticking. After a couple of minutes, flip them over and continue to do this until all sides of the cubes are golden in color. Remove the tofu from the skillet, and if you have any remaining uncooked cubes, cook them now as well.

- Serve the barbecue tofu over the white rice and enjoy!

Tex-Mex Quinoa Salad

This quinoa salad is simple to make, full of nutrients, and delicious! Enjoy it as a full meal either at home or on the road, as it travels well and can be enjoyed either warm or cold.

Chronic Kidney Disease Stage: 1-5/Dialysis

The Details:

The Number of Servings: 2

The Time Needed to Prepare: 5 minutes

The Time Required to Cook: 15 minutes

The Total Preparation/Cook Time: 20 minutes

Number of Calories In Individual Servings: 308

Protein Grams: 8

Phosphorus Milligrams: 252

Potassium Milligrams: 475

Sodium Milligrams: 31

Fat Grams: 12

Total Carbohydrates Grams: 43

Net Carbohydrates Grams: 38

The Ingredients:

- Water – 1 cup
- Olive oil – 1 teaspoon
- Garlic, minced – 2 cloves
- Quinoa, rinsed and drained - .5 cup
- Corn, canned, drained and rinsed - .5 cup
- Bell pepper, chopped - .5
- Green onion, sliced – 2
- Cilantro, fresh, chopped – 2 tablespoons
- Black beans, cooked – .5 cup
- Cumin - .25 teaspoon
- Lime juice – 1.5 tablespoons
- Black pepper, ground - .25 teaspoon
- Chili powder - .5 teaspoon
- Olive oil – 1 tablespoon
- Honey – 1 teaspoon

The Instructions:

1. In a saucepan over medium heat, cook the minced garlic in the single teaspoon of olive oil for one

minute, until fragrant. Add in the water and quinoa and let the pot boiling. Simmer once boiling and cover the pot. Allow the quinoa to cook until all of the liquid has been absorbed, about fifteen minutes. Remove the quinoa from the heat.

1. While the quinoa cooks, prepare the vinaigrette by whisking together the remaining olive oil, honey, lime juice, cumin, chili powder, and black ground pepper.

2. Prepare a big-sized mixing dish where the cooked quinoa can be transferred and toss it together with the prepared vinaigrette, bell pepper, corn, and green onion until it is fully coated. Serve it warm or cold.

Chapter 6: Dinner

In this chapter, you will find recipes perfect for dinner whether you are eating a simple meal for one or a stunning meal for date night. You will love the recipes and how delicious they are.

Shepherd's Pie

This recipe is made with mashed cauliflower instead of potatoes, making it much lower in potassium than traditional Shepherd's pie. Not only that, but it is full of vegetables! In a single serving, you can get nearly half of your daily serving of vegetables.

Chronic Kidney Disease Stage: 1-4

The Details:

The Number of Servings: 2

The Time Needed to Prepare: 5 minutes

The Time Required to Cook: 35 minutes

The Total Preparation/Cook Time: 40 minutes

Number of Calories In Individual Servings: 210

Protein Grams: 14

Phosphorus Milligrams: 192

Potassium Milligrams: 632

Sodium Milligrams: 94

Fat Grams: 11

Total Carbohydrates Grams: 13

Net Carbohydrates Grams: 10

The Ingredients:

- Cauliflower, florets – 2 cups
- Turkey, ground - .25 pound
- Carrots, diced – 1
- Corn kernels - .25 cup
- Celery, diced – stalk
- Poultry seasoning – 1 teaspoon
- Black pepper, ground - .25 teaspoon
- Olive oil - .5 tablespoon

The Instructions:

1. Place in a dish safe for microwave use with some water the cauliflower and cover it with a plate, and

then microwave it until fork-tender. You can also steam it on the stove in a steam basket if you wish.

1. While your cauliflower is steaming, allow the oven to preheat to a Fahrenheit temperature of four-hundred degrees.

2. In a big-sized cooking pot, sauté the celery and carrots in the olive oil for five minutes. Add in the ground turkey and brown it until there is no pink remaining, about nine minutes. Stir in the corn, half of the black pepper, and three-quarters of the poultry seasoning.

3. In a medium-sized kitchen bowl, mash the cauliflower with a hand-held potato masher until it is nice and creamy. Add in the remaining black pepper and poultry seasoning. Set aside the mashed cauliflower.

4. Spread the meat and vegetable mixture into the bottom of a loaf pan. Spread the cauliflower evenly over the top, and then allow it to cook in the preheated oven for twenty minutes. If you want, you can turn the oven's broiler on the last two minutes to get the mashed cauliflower nice and golden.

Italian Herb Chicken and Asparagus

This dish is full of healthy protein from chicken and low in saturated fats. You will love the way that the herbed chicken pairs with the fresh asparagus and mild white rice. Enjoy it for either a high-protein lunch or dinner.

Chronic Kidney Disease Stage: 5/Dialysis

The Details:

The Number of Servings: 2

The Time Needed to Prepare: 5 minutes

The Time Required to Cook: 15 minutes

The Total Preparation/Cook Time: 20 minutes

Number of Calories In Individual Servings: 331

Protein Grams: 22

Phosphorus Milligrams: 259

Potassium Milligrams: 475

Sodium Milligrams: 38

Fat Grams: 9

Total Carbohydrates Grams: 38

Net Carbohydrates Grams: 36

The Ingredients:

- Chicken breast, cut into bite-sized pieces – .33 pound
- Italian herb seasoning – 2 teaspoon
- Black pepper, ground – .25 teaspoon
- Lemon zest - .25 teaspoon
- Garlic, minced – 3 cloves
- Olive oil – 1 tablespoon
- Asparagus, cut into bite-sized pieces - .33 pound
- Rice, white, cooked – 1.5 cups

The Instructions:

1. Preheat your oven to a Fahrenheit temperature of four-hundred and fifty degrees before covering a large sheet pan with kitchen parchment.
1. In a dish that is small in size, toss together the chicken, asparagus, herb seasoning, black pepper, lemon zest, garlic, and olive oil. You want to ensure that all of the ingredients are evenly coated. Either cook this mixture right away or allow it to marinate for fifteen minutes.

2. Place the coated asparagus and chicken onto the baking pan and allow it to cook until the chicken reaches an internal Fahrenheit temperature of one-hundred and sixty-five degrees and the asparagus is tender about fifteen to twenty minutes.

3. Remove the pan from the oven and either immediately serve it over the rice, or store it in the fridge or freezer to enjoy at a later date.

Baked Chicken Tacos

These chicken tacos are simple and easy to cook, as you just fill the tortillas with chicken mixture and then roast them. This gives you a slightly crispy taco shell that is much healthier than the fried alternative.

Chronic Kidney Disease Stage: 1-5/Dialysis

The Details:

The Number of Servings: 2

The Time Needed to Prepare: 5 minutes

The Time Required to Cook: 10 minutes

The Total Preparation/Cook Time: 15 minutes

Number of Calories In Individual Servings: 273

Protein Grams: 24

Phosphorus Milligrams: 423

Potassium Milligrams: 291

Sodium Milligrams: 76

Fat Grams: 9

Total Carbohydrates Grams: 22

Net Carbohydrates Grams: 19

The Ingredients:

- Corn tortillas – 4
- Chicken breast, cooked – 4 ounces
- Cheddar cheese, shredded, low-sodium - .33 cup
- Jalapeno, diced - .5
- Cumin - .25 teaspoon
- Chili powder - .25 teaspoon
- Lime juice – 2 teaspoons

The Instructions:

1. Preheat your oven by setting it to a Fahrenheit temperature of four-hundred degrees. Meanwhile, microwave your tortillas for half a minute so that you can easily work with them without causing them to tear.
1. Either dice the cooked chicken breast with a knife or shred it with a couple of forks. In a mixing dish, place together the cut chicken with the cheese, jalapeno, cumin, chili powder, and lime juice.
2. Set your for tortillas on a baking sheet coated with kitchen parchment, and then fill them with the chicken and cheese mixture. Fold the tortillas in

half, gently pressing them so that they stay folded. Place another baking sheet on top of the tacos, which will both keep them folded during the cooking process and act as an additional heat source to increase the crispiness of the tortilla.

3. Bake the tacos in the preheated oven until they are golden-brown in color, about ten minutes. Watch them carefully, being careful not to allow them to burn.

4. Remove the tacos from the oven immediately and serve them warm, either plain or with Greek yogurt in place of sour cream.

Mushroom Kale Quesadillas

These quesadillas are simple and easy to make and taste delicious! You will love the way that the mushrooms and kale perfectly complement the creamy cheese.

Chronic Kidney Disease Stage: 1-5/Dialysis

The Details:

The Number of Servings: 2

The Time Needed to Prepare: 5 minutes

The Time Required to Cook: 15 minutes

The Total Preparation/Cook Time: 20 minutes

Number of Calories In Individual Servings: 305

Protein Grams: 14

Phosphorus Milligrams: 462

Potassium Milligrams: 595

Sodium Milligrams: 24

Fat Grams: 15

Total Carbohydrates Grams: 30

Net Carbohydrates Grams: 26

The Ingredients:

- Tortillas, low-sodium, 8 inch – 4
- Olive oil – 1 tablespoon
- Mushrooms, sliced – 8 ounces
- Mozzarella cheese, shredded, low-sodium - .25 cup
- Cheddar cheese, shredded, low-sodium - .25 cup
- Kale, chopped – 3 cups

The Instructions:

- Preheat your oven by setting it to a Fahrenheit temperature of four-hundred degrees and prepare a baking sheet by lining it with kitchen parchment.
- Place the sliced mushrooms in a microwave-safe bowl and then soften them by cooking them in the microwave for three minutes. Drain off any liquid and then set them aside.
- Using a pastry brush, coat both sides of all the tortillas with the olive oil, and then set two of them on the prepared baking sheet. Over both of the tortillas on the baking sheet divide the sliced mushrooms, kale, mozzarella cheese, and cheddar

cheese. Place the remaining two tortillas on top of this mixture.

- Place a baking sheet on top of the quesadillas and then place the two trays in the oven for twelve minutes, until the tortilla is golden and the cheese has melted. Remove the quesadillas from the oven, slice them up, and serve them alone or with a dollop of Greek yogurt.

Creamy Italian Chicken

This creamy dish is made healthy by using Greek yogurt in place of heavy cream, but it is still full of flavor thanks to the garlic and Parmesan cheese. Enjoy this chicken alongside your favorite grains and vegetables for a full meal.

Chronic Kidney Disease Stage: 1-5/Dialysis

The Details:

The Number of Servings: 2

The Time Needed to Prepare: 5 minutes

The Time Required to Cook: 15 minutes

The Total Preparation/Cook Time: 20 minutes

Number of Calories In Individual Servings: 225

Protein Grams: 20

Phosphorus Milligrams: 270

Potassium Milligrams: 419

Sodium Milligrams: 268

Fat Grams: 12

Total Carbohydrates Grams: 7

Net Carbohydrates Grams: 6

The Ingredients:

- Chicken breast, thinly sliced – 4 ounces
- Greek yogurt, plain - .25 cup
- Olive oil – 1 tablespoon
- Italian seasoning - .5 teaspoon
- Garlic powder - .5 teaspoon
- Parmesan cheese, grated - .25 cup
- Kale, chopped - .5 cup
- Bell pepper, thinly sliced – 1
- Water – 3 tablespoons

The Instructions:

1. Into a large skillet, add the sliced chicken and olive oil over medium heat, cooking the slices until cooked through and golden brown, about seven to ten minutes. The internal temperature of the chicken must reach Fahrenheit one-hundred and sixty-five degrees.

1. Remove the chicken from the pan and set it aside on a plate. Meanwhile, place the thinly sliced bell pepper, kale, Parmesan cheese, garlic powder, Italian seasoning, water, and the Greek yogurt into

the pan. Cook this until the cheese is melted, it is warm, and just reaches a simmer.

2. Place the chicken back into the simmering sauce and allow it to cook in the sauce for one minute before removing the dish from the heat.

Chicken and Rice Scampi

This chicken and rice scampi are creamy and full of flavor! It includes white wine, and the alcohol is cooked off during the cooking process. However, if you don't want to use white wine, you can use extra low-sodium chicken broth in its place.

Chronic Kidney Disease Stage: 1-5/Dialysis

The Details:

The Number of Servings: 2

The Time Needed to Prepare: 5 minutes

The Time Required to Cook: 15 minutes

The Total Preparation/Cook Time: 20 minutes

Number of Calories In Individual Servings: 403

Protein Grams: 20

Phosphorus Milligrams: 255

Potassium Milligrams: 324

Sodium Milligrams: 233

Fat Grams: 18

Total Carbohydrates Grams: 37

Net Carbohydrates Grams: 37

The Ingredients:

- Chicken breast, thinly sliced – 4 ounces
- Olive oil – 1 tablespoon
- Garlic powder - .25 teaspoon
- Black pepper, ground - .25 teaspoon
- Butter – 2 tablespoons
- Garlic, minced – 1 tablespoon
- Red pepper flakes - .25 teaspoon
- White wine, dry – 3 tablespoons
- White rice, cooked – 1.5 cup
- Parmesan cheese, grated – 3 tablespoons
- Greek yogurt, plain – 2 tablespoons
- Chicken broth, low-sodium – 3 tablespoons

The Instructions:

1. Season your sliced chicken with the garlic powder and black ground pepper. Then, place it in a large skillet over medium heat along with the olive oil.
1. Allow the chicken to sauté until it is cooked through and seared, about eight minutes. The internal temperature of the chicken must reach

Fahrenheit one-hundred and sixty-five degrees. Remove the chicken from the skillet and set it aside on a plate.

2. Add the butter, red pepper flakes, and minced garlic, and allow the garlic to cook for three minutes. Stir in the Greek yogurt, white wine, and chicken broth, stirring the mixture completely and allowing it to simmer for five minutes.

3. Stir in the Parmesan cheese and place the chicken back in the pan, allowing it to simmer in the sauce for one minute.

4. Remove the skillet from the heat and serve the chicken and sauce over the cooked white rice while still warm.

Mushroom Parmesan Pasta

With this creamy mushroom and Parmesan pasta dish, you won't miss traditional tomato sauces in the slightest! This sauce is much lower in potassium and phosphorus, but even more delicious. Enjoy this pasta alone, or with a side of homemade garlic bread.

Chronic Kidney Disease Stage: 1-5/Dialysis

The Details:

The Number of Servings: 2

The Time Needed to Prepare: 5 minutes

The Time Required to Cook: 15 minutes

The Total Preparation/Cook Time: 20 minutes

Number of Calories In Individual Servings: 398

Protein Grams: 14

Phosphorus Milligrams: 235

Potassium Milligrams: 374

Sodium Milligrams: 124

Fat Grams: 16

Total Carbohydrates Grams: 48

Net Carbohydrates Grams: 46

The Ingredients:

- Bowtie pasta – 4 ounces
- Olive oil – 2 tablespoons
- Mushrooms, sliced – 1 cup
- Garlic, minced – 1 tablespoon
- Onion, diced - .25 cup
- Chicken broth, low-sodium - .5 cup
- Greek yogurt, plain - .25 cup
- Parmesan cheese – 2 tablespoons
- Black pepper, ground - .25 teaspoon
- Kale, chopped – 1 cup

The Instructions:

1. Bring a pot of water to a boil and cook the pasta according to the directions on the package. Drain off the pasta water and set the pasta aside.
1. While the pasta cooks, in a large skillet, cook together the mushrooms, onions, and garlic in the olive oil until the mushrooms are soft and golden, about five to seven minutes. Add in the Greek yogurt, kale, black pepper, Parmesan cheese, and chicken broth. Cook the mixture for five more

minutes until the kale is wilted and the sauce is simmering.

2. Toss together the pasta and the mushroom sauce, and then serve the dish immediately.

Stuffed Bell Pepper Soup

This soup is simple to make and delicious! You will love the stuffed bell pepper flavor, but made with much more ease. This soup is easy to cook and only tastes better once it has a chance to chill in the fridge overnight allowing the flavors to meld. That means you can enjoy one serving for dinner and enjoy another serving from lunch the following day.

Chronic Kidney Disease Stage: 1-5/Dialysis

The Details:

The Number of Servings: 2

The Time Needed to Prepare: 5 minutes

The Time Required to Cook: 20 minutes

The Total Preparation/Cook Time: 25 minutes

Number of Calories In Individual Servings: 283

Protein Grams: 16

Phosphorus Milligrams: 183

Potassium Milligrams: 369

Sodium Milligrams: 85

Fat Grams: 9

Total Carbohydrates Grams: 32

Net Carbohydrates Grams: 30

The Ingredients:

- Chicken broth, low-sodium – 2 cups
- Bell pepper, red, diced – 1
- Garlic, minced – 4 cloves
- Onion, diced - .5 cup
- Ground turkey – 4 ounces
- Olive oil – 2 teaspoons
- Italian seasoning – 1 teaspoon
- White rice, cooked – 1 cup
- Parsley, fresh, chopped – 1 tablespoon

The Instructions:

1. In a large pan over medium heat, cook the ground turkey with the olive oil, onion, and garlic until the turkey is fully cooked and no pink is remaining about five to seven minutes.
1. Add the black pepper, Italian seasoning, and bell pepper to the soup pot, allowing it to cook for three more minutes.

2. Into the pot, pour the low-sodium chicken broth, simmer the soup for fifteen minutes, until the bell peppers are tender. Stir in the cooked rice and parsley before serving.

Seared Chicken and Green Beans

This chicken is delicious and simple to make, and it perfectly pairs with the fresh lemon green beans. Enjoy this chicken alongside your favorite grains for a complete meal.

Chronic Kidney Disease Stage: 1-5/Dialysis

The Details:

The Number of Servings: 2

The Time Needed to Prepare: 5 minutes

The Time Required to Cook: 15 minutes

The Total Preparation/Cook Time: 20 minutes

Number of Calories In Individual Servings: 160

Protein Grams: 14

Phosphorus Milligrams: 156

Potassium Milligrams: 385

Sodium Milligrams: 37

Fat Grams: 8

Total Carbohydrates Grams: 7

Net Carbohydrates Grams: 5

The Ingredients:

- Chicken breast – 4 ounces
- Green beans, trimmed – .25 pound
- Garlic, minced – 3 cloves
- Olive oil – 1 tablespoon
- Paprika - .25 teaspoon
- Onion powder - .25 teaspoon
- Black pepper, ground - .25 teaspoon
- Lemon juice – 1 tablespoon
- Chicken broth, low-sodium – 2 tablespoons
- Water - .25 cup
- Red chili flakes - .25 teaspoon
- Parsley, fresh, chopped – 3 tablespoons

The Instructions:

1. Season the chicken with the onion powder, black pepper, and paprika, and then set it aside.
1. Meanwhile, place the green beans in a microwave-safe bowl along with the water. Steam the green beans in the microwave for eight minutes until they are almost cooked but still a little crisp.

2. In a large skillet, cook the seasoned chicken in the olive oil until it is cooked all the way through, about seven to ten minutes. The chicken is only done cooking once it reaches an internal Fahrenheit temperature of one-hundred and sixty-five degrees. Remove the chicken from the skillet and set it aside.

3. Into the skillet add the garlic, parsley, chili flakes, and the microwaved green beans. Allow them to cook for an additional four minutes until they are tender to your preference. Add in the lemon juice, chicken broth, and cooked chicken, allowing the sauce to simmer for two to three minutes.

4. Remove the skillet from the heat and serve immediately with a side of grains or bread.

Poached Thai Salmon

This poached salmon is full of Thai flavors such as lemongrass, ginger, and garlic. You will love the flavor, especially when it is served with freshly cooked rice. Try topping the rice with a little extra lime juice for added flavor.

Chronic Kidney Disease Stage: 1-5/Dialysis

The Details:

The Number of Servings: 2

The Time Needed to Prepare: 5 minutes

The Time Required to Cook: 15 minutes

The Total Preparation/Cook Time: 20 minutes

Number of Calories In Individual Servings: 250

Protein Grams: 18

Phosphorus Milligrams: 257

Potassium Milligrams: 446

Sodium Milligrams: 108

Fat Grams: 16

Total Carbohydrates Grams: 8

Net Carbohydrates Grams: 7

The Ingredients:

- Salmon fillets – 6 ounces
- Black pepper, ground - .25 teaspoon
- Olive oil – 1 tablespoon
- Garlic, minced – 2 cloves
- Ginger powder – 1 teaspoon
- Lemongrass, peeled and grated – 1 tablespoon
- Brown sugar – 2 teaspoons
- Red chili flakes – 1 teaspoon
- Coconut milk – 3 tablespoons
- Lime juice – 2 teaspoons
- Lime zest - .25 teaspoon

The Instructions:

1. Season the salmon with the black pepper and then sear it in a skillet over medium-high heat in the olive oil. Cook the salmon skin-side up at first, then after one to two minutes, flip it over and cook the skin-side down for one minute. Remove the salmon from the skillet and place it on a plate.

1. Reduce the heat of the skillet to medium-low and add in the lemongrass and garlic, allowing them to cook until golden, about one minute. Add in the sugar, ground ginger, and red pepper flakes, about thirty seconds until caramelized.

2. Stir in the coconut milk, deglazing the pan in the process. Add the salmon back into the sauce and allow it to gently simmer until cooked, about four minutes.

3. Add the lime juice and zest to the skillet, and serve it with either rice or noodles.

The Best Turkey Burgers

These burgers are not only delicious, but they are also incredibly simple! You can serve them alongside a bed of rice, wrapped in lettuce, with store-bought low-sodium buns, or you can even make your own buns. Try turning the Fluffy Sandwich Bread or the French Bread from later on in this book into hamburger buns and you will not be disappointed!

Chronic Kidney Disease Stage: 1-5/Dialysis

The Details:

The Number of Servings: 2

The Time Needed to Prepare: 5 minutes

The Time Required to Cook: 15 minutes

The Total Preparation/Cook Time: 20 minutes

Number of Calories In Individual Servings: 130

Protein Grams: 11

Phosphorus Milligrams: 129

Potassium Milligrams: 206

Sodium Milligrams: 37

Fat Grams: 8

Total Carbohydrates Grams: 3

Net Carbohydrates Grams: 3

The Ingredients:

- Turkey, ground - .25 pound
- Garlic, minced – 2 cloves
- Onion, diced - .25 cup
- Parsley, fresh, chopped – 2 tablespoons
- Mustard seed, ground - .25 teaspoon
- Red pepper flakes - .25 teaspoon
- Black pepper, ground - .125 teaspoon
- Olive oil - .5 tablespoon

The Instructions:

1. In a bowl, lightly knead together the ground turkey, onion, garlic, parsley, and spices. Be careful to not over mix the meat, otherwise, it becomes tough. You only want to mix it just until combined.
1. Use your hands to form the meat into two patties of even thickness. You want to make them slightly larger than the buns since the meat will shrink as it cooks.

2. Grease a skillet with the olive oil and pan fry the patties over medium heat until they are cooked through with an internal temperature of one-hundred and sixty-five degrees Fahrenheit. You can also cook them under your oven's broiler or on the grill for the best flavor.

Chapter 7: Side Dishes

These side dishes can complement any meal. Whether you have made an elaborate entree or are eating a simple slice of chicken, you can enjoy these side dishes to both increase the flavor and the nutrition. You will find both grain and vegetable-based side dishes in this chapter, ensuring that you have something for every occasion.

Lime Cilantro Rice

Rice is a wonderful way to bulk up your meals and add needed calories, without adding too much excess phosphorus, potassium, or sodium. This rice is particularly tasty, as it is full of lime and cilantro, making it a wonderful option whenever you want to enjoy a fresh dish or Tex-Mex.

Chronic Kidney Disease Stage: 1-5/Dialysis

The Details:

The Number of Servings: 2

The Time Needed to Prepare: 5 minutes

The Time Required to Cook: 20 minutes

The Total Preparation/Cook Time: 25 minutes

Number of Calories In Individual Servings: 363

Protein Grams: 5

Phosphorus Milligrams: 74

Potassium Milligrams: 86

Sodium Milligrams: 5

Fat Grams: 10

Total Carbohydrates Grams: 60

Net Carbohydrates Grams: 58

The Ingredients:

- White rice – .75 cup
- Water – 1.5 cups
- Olive oil – 1.5 tablespoons
- Bay leaf, ground - .25 teaspoon
- Lime juice – 1 tablespoon
- Lemon juice – 1 tablespoon
- Lime zest - .25 teaspoon
- Cilantro, chopped - .25 cup

The Instructions:

1. Place the white rice and water in a medium-sized saucepan and bring it to a boil over medium heat. Reduce the heat to a light simmer and cover the pot with a lid, allowing it to cook until all of the water has been absorbed about eighteen to twenty minutes.

1. Once the rice is done cooking, stir in the ground bay leaf, olive oil, lime juice, lemon juice, lime zest, and cilantro. You want to do this with a fork, preferably, as this will fluff the rice rather than causing it to compact. Serve while warm.

Spanish Rice

Unlike most Spanish rice, this one does not contain tomatoes. However, it is still high on flavors and you will find it is the perfect addition for tacos, burritos, and simply as a side dish whenever you crave a burst of flavor.

Chronic Kidney Disease Stage: 1-5/Dialysis

The Details:

The Number of Servings: 2

The Time Needed to Prepare: 5 minutes

The Time Required to Cook: 20 minutes

The Total Preparation/Cook Time: 25 minutes

Number of Calories In Individual Servings: 303

Protein Grams: 6

Phosphorus Milligrams: 104

Potassium Milligrams: 197

Sodium Milligrams: 57

Fat Grams: 1

Total Carbohydrates Grams: 65

Net Carbohydrates Grams: 63

The Ingredients:

- White rice – .75 cup
- Chicken broth, low sodium – 1.5 cups
- Onion dehydrated flakes – 2 tablespoons
- Garlic, minced – 2 cloves
- Lemon juice – 1 tablespoon
- Cumin, ground - .25 teaspoon
- Chili powder - .5 teaspoon
- Oregano, dried - .5 teaspoon
- Black pepper, ground - .25 teaspoon
- Cilantro, chopped – 3 tablespoons

The Instructions:

1. Place the rice, chicken broth, onion flakes, and minced garlic in a medium-sized saucepan. Bring the chicken broth and rice to a boil over medium heat, and then reduce the heat to a light simmer, cover it with a lid, and allow it to cook until the liquid has all been absorbed about eighteen to twenty minutes.//
1. Use a fork to fluff the rice mix in the lemon juice, cumin, chili powder, oregano, black pepper, and cilantro. Once combined, serve the rice while still warm.

Parmesan Quinoa with Peas

This Parmesan quinoa might be higher in minerals than rice dishes, however, if you have a little extra room for phosphorus and potassium in your daily allotment, you will love the addition of this dish! This dish is great when you need a little extra protein, or simply want an easy side dish that feels fancy.

Chronic Kidney Disease Stage: 1-5/Dialysis

The Details:

The Number of Servings: 2

The Time Needed to Prepare: 5 minutes

The Time Required to Cook: 20 minutes

The Total Preparation/Cook Time: 25 minutes

Number of Calories In Individual Servings: 386

Protein Grams: 13

Phosphorus Milligrams: 378

Potassium Milligrams: 465

Sodium Milligrams: 144

Fat Grams: 16

Total Carbohydrates Grams: 47

Net Carbohydrates Grams: 41

The Ingredients:

- Quinoa – .75 cup
- Water – 1.5 cups
- Green peas, thawed if frozen - .75 cup
- Black pepper, ground - .25 teaspoon
- Olive oil – 1.5 tablespoons
- Parmesan cheese, grated – 3 tablespoons

The Instructions:

1. Place the uncooked quinoa in a fine metal sieve and rinse it well with water until there is no debris running off.

1. Place the quinoa and water in a medium-sized metal saucepan and bring it to a boil over medium heat. Once it attains a boil, reduce it to a light simmer, cover the pot with a lid, and allow it to cook until the water has all been absorbed. This should take fifteen to twenty minutes.

2. Remove the quinoa from the heat and allow it to sit with the lid on for five minutes. Once it has set, use a fork to fluff the quinoa and stir in the green

peas, olive oil, and quinoa. Close the lid once again, allowing it to sit for five additional minutes to warm the peas and melt the cheese. Enjoy the quinoa while warm.

Mushroom Orzo

Orzo is a type of pasta formed in the shape of rice. It has a wonderful flavor and texture, and due to the small sizes, it greatly absorbs the flavor of whatever it is cooked. You will love this orzo with the addition of mushrooms, garlic, and sage.

Chronic Kidney Disease Stage: 1-5/Dialysis

The Details:

The Number of Servings: 2

The Time Needed to Prepare: 5 minutes

The Time Required to Cook: 20 minutes

The Total Preparation/Cook Time: 25 minutes

Number of Calories In Individual Servings: 337

Protein Grams: 18

Phosphorus Milligrams: 63

Potassium Milligrams: 430

Sodium Milligrams: 43

Fat Grams: 8

Total Carbohydrates Grams: 99

Net Carbohydrates Grams: 95

The Ingredients:

- Orzo - .75 cup
- Chicken broth, low-sodium – 1.25 cup
- Mushrooms, diced – 4 ounces
- Garlic, minced – 3 cloves
- Onion flakes, dehydrated – 1 tablespoon
- Olive oil – 1 tablespoon
- Sage, ground - .25 teaspoon

The Instructions:

1. Place the diced mushrooms, olive oil, and garlic in a medium-sized metal saucepan and allow them to sauté over medium heat for five minutes. Add in the sage, onion flakes, orzo, and low-sodium chicken broth. Bring the mixture to a boil.//
1. Reduce the heat of the skillet to a light simmer, cover the pot with a lid, and allow it to cook until all of the liquid has been absorbed about nine minutes. Fluff the orzo with a fork before serving.

Carrot and Pineapple Slaw

This slaw is sweet and savory with the pineapple and grapes perfectly complementing the carrots. You will especially love that this slaw can be made up to a day in advance, making it the perfect side dish to take with you to work, on a road trip, or to a potluck.

Chronic Kidney Disease Stage: 1-5/Dialysis

The Details:

The Number of Servings: 2

The Time Needed to Prepare: 5 minutes

The Time Required to Cook: 0 minutes

The Total Preparation/Cook Time: 5 minutes

Number of Calories In Individual Servings: 264

Protein Grams: 2

Phosphorus Milligrams: 74

Potassium Milligrams: 423

Sodium Milligrams: 91

Fat Grams: 17

Total Carbohydrates Grams: 29

Net Carbohydrates Grams: 25

The Ingredients:

- Carrot matchsticks – 5 ounces
- Pineapple chunks, canned, liquid drained - .5 cup
- Grapes, sliced in half - .5 cup
- Pecan pieces - .25 cup
- Mayonnaise, low-sodium - .33 cup
- Lemon juice – 1 tablespoon

The Instructions:

1. In a bowl, toss together the carrot matchsticks, drained pineapple chunks, sliced grapes, and pecan pieces. Stir in the low-sodium mayonnaise and lemon juice.
1. Cover the bowl with plastic wrap or a lid and then allow it to chill and marinate for at least an hour before serving. You can make this slaw up to a day in advance.

Sesame Cucumber Salad

This is a take on a popular dish throughout East Asia, although this version does not use soy sauce which is high in sodium and other minerals. However, this salad is still full of flavor, making it the perfect refreshing dish to enjoy in the summer months.

Chronic Kidney Disease Stage: 1-5/Dialysis

The Details:

The Number of Servings: 2

The Time Needed to Prepare: 5 minutes

The Time Required to Cook: 0 minutes

The Total Preparation/Cook Time: 5 minutes

Number of Calories In Individual Servings: 92

Protein Grams: 1

Phosphorus Milligrams: 46

Potassium Milligrams: 250

Sodium Milligrams: 117

Fat Grams: 5

Total Carbohydrates Grams: 9

Net Carbohydrates Grams: 8

The Ingredients:

- Cucumbers, thinly sliced – 1
- Sesame seeds - .5 teaspoon
- Rice wine vinegar – 1 tablespoon
- Sugar - .5 tablespoon
- Sesame seed oil – 1.5 tablespoons
- Red pepper flakes - .25 teaspoon

The Instructions:

1. You want the cucumbers sliced as thinly as you can get them. While you can certainly do this with a knife, it is quicker and easier if you use a mandolin.
1. In a medium to a small bowl, whisk together the sesame seeds, rice wine vinegar, sugar, sesame seed oil, and red pepper flakes. Once well combined, add in the cucumbers and toss the vegetables in the vinaigrette. Serve immediately.

Creamy Jalapeno Corn

This creamy jalapeno corn is the perfect treat for the summer, especially when paired with grilled foods. Try this corn alongside grilled chicken or turkey burgers, and you will absolutely love it!

Chronic Kidney Disease Stage: 1-5/Dialysis

The Details:

The Number of Servings: 2

The Time Needed to Prepare: 5 minutes

The Time Required to Cook: 15 minutes

The Total Preparation/Cook Time: 20 minutes

Number of Calories In Individual Servings: 284

Protein Grams: 7

Phosphorus Milligrams: 200

Potassium Milligrams: 293

Sodium Milligrams: 82

Fat Grams: 19

Total Carbohydrates Grams: 20

Net Carbohydrates Grams: 18

The Ingredients:

- Corn kernels, fresh – 1 cup
- Red bell pepper, diced - .25 cup
- Jalapeno, seeded and diced – 1
- Cream cheese – 1.5 ounces
- Olive oil – 1 tablespoon
- Black pepper, ground - .25 teaspoon
- Cheddar cheese, low-sodium - .25 cup

The Instructions:

1. Preheat your oven to a Fahrenheit temperature of three-hundred and fifty degrees.//
1. In a medium saucepan, sauté the bell pepper and jalapeno in the olive oil until softened, about four minutes. Add in the cream cheese and continue to stir until it melts and combines with the vegetables.
2. Add in the corn, black pepper, and half of the cheese. After the mixture is combined, sprinkle the remaining cheese over the top and place the saucepan in the oven to cook until it is hot and bubbling about fifteen minutes.

Crispy Parmesan Cauliflower

This cauliflower is coated in Parmesan cheese and breadcrumbs for a flavorful and crispy coating, allowing you to enjoy a savory treat. If you are someone who has a weakness for French fries, you will also love this cauliflower.

Chronic Kidney Disease Stage: 1-5/Dialysis

The Details:

The Number of Servings: 2

The Time Needed to Prepare: 5 minutes

The Time Required to Cook: 30 minutes

The Total Preparation/Cook Time: 35 minutes

Number of Calories In Individual Servings: 106

Protein Grams: 5

Phosphorus Milligrams: 166

Potassium Milligrams: 369

Sodium Milligrams: 222

Fat Grams: 9

Total Carbohydrates Grams: 16

Net Carbohydrates Grams: 14

The Ingredients:

- Cauliflower florets – 2 cups
- Black pepper, ground - .125 teaspoon
- Garlic, minced – 2 cloves
- Parmesan cheese, grated – 2 tablespoons
- Bread crumbs, plain - .25 cup
- Olive oil – 1 tablespoon

The Instructions:

1. Preheat your oven to a Fahrenheit temperature of four-hundred degrees and line a baking sheet with kitchen parchment.
1. In one small bowl, combine the olive oil and the garlic. In another, combine the Parmesan cheese, bread crumbs, and black pepper.
2. Dip the cauliflower piece-by-piece first into the olive oil mixture, and then into the bread crumb mixture. After you coat each piece, set it on the kitchen parchment-lined sheet.
3. Place the cauliflower sheet in the middle of the oven and roast the cauliflower until it reaches golden brown perfection, about thirty minutes. Serve it immediately, while it is still warm and crispy.

Cucumber Dill Salad with Greek Yogurt Dressing

This creamy dill salad is full of refreshing flavors, making it ideal to enjoy alongside savory meals. Whether you are eating a light meal of fish or a heavier meal, you will find that this salad with the fresh dill and zesty Greek yogurt complements anything savory.

Chronic Kidney Disease Stage: 1-5/Dialysis

The Details:

The Number of Servings: 2

The Time Needed to Prepare: 5 minutes

The Time Required to Cook: 0 minutes

The Total Preparation/Cook Time: 5 minutes

Number of Calories In Individual Servings: 106

Protein Grams: 5

Phosphorus Milligrams: 166

Potassium Milligrams: 369

Sodium Milligrams: 222

Fat Grams: 9

Total Carbohydrates Grams: 16

Net Carbohydrates Grams: 14

The Ingredients:

- Cucumbers, cut thinly – 2
- Red onion, small, thinly sliced - .5
- Greek yogurt, plain – 3 tablespoons
- Honey – 2 teaspoons
- White vinegar – 4 teaspoons
- Black pepper, ground - .125 teaspoon
- Garlic powder - .125 teaspoon
- Dill, fresh, chopped – 1.5 tablespoons

The Instructions:

1. Use either a knife or a mandolin to cut the cucumbers into thin and even slices, about .25 of an inch thick.
1. In a medium bowl, whisk together the fresh dill, garlic powder, black pepper, white vinegar, honey, and Greek yogurt.
2. Into the bowl with the prepared Greek yogurt dressing, add the cucumbers and red onion, and toss them together until fully coated. Cover the bowl with a lid or plastic wrap and allow it to chill in the fridge for at least an hour before enjoying. You can make this salad up to a day in advance.

<u>Zesty Green Beans with Almonds</u>

These green beans are full of flavor from zesty lemon, shallot, and garlic, which is perfectly complemented by the nutty and creamy sliced almonds. These green beans may be simple, but they feel extraordinary.

Chronic Kidney Disease Stage: 1-5/Dialysis

The Details:

The Number of Servings: 2

The Time Needed to Prepare: 5 minutes

The Time Required to Cook: 10 minutes

The Total Preparation/Cook Time: 15 minutes

Number of Calories In Individual Servings: 143

Protein Grams: 3

Phosphorus Milligrams: 84

Potassium Milligrams: 322

Sodium Milligrams: 8

Fat Grams: 10

Total Carbohydrates Grams: 11

Net Carbohydrates Grams: 8

The Ingredients:

- Green beans, trimmed - .5 pound
- Olive oil – 1 tablespoon
- Shallot, diced – 1
- Garlic, minced – 2 cloves
- Almonds, sliced – 2 tablespoons
- Lemon zest - .25 teaspoon
- Lemon juice – 1 teaspoon
- Black pepper, ground - .125 teaspoon

The Instructions:

1. In a large skillet, sauté the shallot and garlic in the olive oil over medium heat until soft, about three minutes. Add in the green beans and black pepper and continue to cook the green beans until they are tender about seven minutes.//
1. Once the green beans are ready, stir in the lemon juice and lemon zest, and then top the skillet off with the sliced almonds.

Roasted Carrots and Broccoli

These vegetables are roasted to perfection, allowing you to enjoy the sweet and savory pair of carrots and broccoli. These vegetables are not only full of flavor but also nutrients, making them a wonderful choice to add to your meal plan.

Chronic Kidney Disease Stage: 1-5/Dialysis

The Details:

The Number of Servings: 2

The Time Needed to Prepare: 5 minutes

The Time Required to Cook: 20 minutes

The Total Preparation/Cook Time: 25 minutes

Number of Calories In Individual Servings: 184

Protein Grams: 4

Phosphorus Milligrams: 100

Potassium Milligrams: 494

Sodium Milligrams: 86

Fat Grams: 14

Total Carbohydrates Grams: 12

Net Carbohydrates Grams: 8

The Ingredients:

- Broccoli Florets - .5 pound
- Carrot, large, cut on the bias – 1
- Olive oil – 2 tablespoons
- Garlic, minced – 2 cloves
- Lemon zest - .5 tablespoon
- Parmesan cheese – .5 tablespoon
- Lemon juice - .5 tablespoon
- Black pepper, ground - .125 teaspoon

The Instructions:

- Preheat your oven to a Fahrenheit temperature of four-hundred and fifty degrees.
- In a bowl, toss together the black pepper, garlic, olive oil, chopped carrot, and broccoli florets. Spread the vegetable mixture onto a baking sheet.
- Roast the vegetables until they are tender and lightly browned, about fifteen to twenty minutes. Remove the pan from the stove, transfer them back to the bowl from earlier, and toss them with the lemon zest, lemon juice, and grated Parmesan cheese. Enjoy the vegetables while still warm.

Tahini and Pomegranate Carrots

These carrots are extravagant enough to enjoy on Thanksgiving or Christmas, but easy enough to cook any day of the week. Enjoy these carrots whether you wish to wow a crowd or enjoy a rich and flavorful treat.

Chronic Kidney Disease Stage: 1-5/Dialysis

The Details:

The Number of Servings: 2

The Time Needed to Prepare: 5 minutes

The Time Required to Cook: 30 minutes

The Total Preparation/Cook Time: 35 minutes

Number of Calories In Individual Servings: 143

Protein Grams: 2

Phosphorus Milligrams: 102

Potassium Milligrams: 434

Sodium Milligrams: 88

Fat Grams: 9

Total Carbohydrates Grams: 14

Net Carbohydrates Grams: 10

The Ingredients:

- Carrots - .5 pound
- Olive oil – 2 teaspoons
- Tahini paste – 1 tablespoon
- Cilantro, chopped – 1 tablespoon
- Cumin seeds - .5 teaspoon
- Black pepper, ground - .125 teaspoon
- Pomegranate arils – 2 tablespoons

The Instructions:

- Set the oven to a Fahrenheit temperature of three-hundred and seventy-five.
- In a bowl, toss together the whole carrots with the olive oil, cumin seeds, and black pepper. Place them on a baking sheet and allow them to roast until tender, about thirty minutes.
- Remove the carrots from the oven and drizzle the tahini over them, and then sprinkle both the cilantro and the pomegranate arils over the top before serving.

Chapter 8: Breads

In this chapter, you will find all the breads your heart might wish for. Unlike the breads commonly sold on the market, these are all low-sodium, allowing you to enjoy them to your heart's content. Whether you are craving something savory or sweet, you are sure to find what you wish for here.

<u>Fluffy Sandwich Bread</u>

This bread is perfect for sandwiches, as it is light, fluffy, and rich. Not only is it good for sandwiches, but you can also enjoy it for breakfast as toast.

Chronic Kidney Disease Stage: 1-5/Dialysis

The Details:

The Number of Servings: 5

The Time Needed to Prepare: 15 minutes

The Time Required to Cook: 30 minutes

The Total Preparation/Cook Time: 45 minutes

Number of Calories In Individual Servings: 371

Protein Grams: 8

Phosphorus Milligrams: 95

Potassium Milligrams: 122

Sodium Milligrams: 45

Fat Grams: 8

Total Carbohydrates Grams: 64

Net Carbohydrates Grams: 62

The Ingredients:

- Almond milk, warm – 1 cup
- Olive oil – 2 tablespoons
- Honey – 1 tablespoon
- Active dry yeast – 1 packet
- All-purpose flour – 3 cups
- Butter, melted – 1 tablespoon

The Instructions:

1. Place the milk, honey, and yeast into the bowl of your stand mixer, whisking them together until the yeast is completely dissolved. Allow this to sit in a warm place for five to ten minutes, until the yeast is especially foamy and bubbly.

1. Once the yeast is bubbly, add in the all-purpose flour and olive oil. Add the hook attachment onto your stand mixer and knead the dough until it is smooth and pulls away from the sides of the bowl, about ten minutes. Be sure that the stand mixer is on low speed.

2. Cover the bowl of the stand mixer with a clean kitchen towel, and allow it to rise in a warm place until it doubles in size, about an hour.

3. Once the dough has risen, punch it down and place it in a loaf pan, greased with olive oil. Cover this pan back up with the clean towel and allow it to rise once more in a warm location until doubled in size, about forty-five minutes.

4. Bake your risen bread loaf in an oven preheated to three-hundred and twenty-five degrees until it is cooked through, about twenty-five to thirty minutes. Once the loaf is removed from the oven, use a pastry brush and coat the top of the loaf with melted butter.

No-Knead Rustic Loaf

This loaf is incredibly simple, yet resembles the rustic gourmet loaves from Italy and France. Enjoy this loaf as a simple sandwich, grilled panini, morning toast, or even to make bread crumbs to cook with.

Chronic Kidney Disease Stage: 1-5/Dialysis

The Details:

The Number of Servings: 4

The Time Needed to Prepare: 10 minutes

The Time Required to Cook: 45 minutes

The Total Preparation/Cook Time: 55 minutes

Number of Calories In Individual Servings: 346

Protein Grams: 10

Phosphorus Milligrams: 111

Potassium Milligrams: 115

Sodium Milligrams: 4

Fat Grams: 1

Total Carbohydrates Grams: 72

Net Carbohydrates Grams: 70

The Ingredients:

- All-purpose flour – 3 cups
- Active dry yeast – 1.5 teaspoons
- Water, warm – 1.5 cups

The Instructions:

1. In a large bowl, combine the flour and yeast, and then add the flour and combine it with a spoon until it forms a thick dough. This dough will likely stick to the bottom of the bowl which is okay.

1. Cover your bowl with a clean kitchen towel, and allow it to rise in a warm location until doubled about two to three hours.

2. Set your oven to a Fahrenheit temperature of four-hundred and fifty degrees. While you can use a standard aluminum pan; if you have a pizza stone, you can set this in the oven to warm for forty-five minutes before using. Fill a small dish with two inches of water and place it at the bottom of your oven. Don't skip this step, as the steam from the water creates a crispy crust.

3. Sprinkle some flour onto a clean cutting board and place your bread loaf on it. Use your hands to form

the bread into a round ball, without kneading. Use a sharp knife and score the top of the load with a large knife.

4. Place the dough onto the hot pizza stone or a prepared aluminum pan and place it in the oven to cook until golden brown, crisp, and cooked through, about forty-five minutes. Once done cooking, allow the loaf to cool completely before cutting.

Pita Bread

Whereas pita bread you buy in the store can contain a decent amount of sodium, this homemade pita bread only contains three milligrams! That means you can enjoy pita as much as you would like, allowing you to make simple sandwiches or more complex Indian meals.

Chronic Kidney Disease Stage: 1-5/Dialysis

The Details:

The Number of Servings: 4

The Time Needed to Prepare: 30 minutes

The Time Required to Cook: 30 minutes

The Total Preparation/Cook Time: 60 minutes

Number of Calories In Individual Servings: 272

Protein Grams: 8

Phosphorus Milligrams: 91

Potassium Milligrams: 97

Sodium Milligrams: 3

Fat Grams: 0

Total Carbohydrates Grams: 56

Net Carbohydrates Grams: 54

The Ingredients:

- All-purpose flour – 3.5 cups
- Water, warm – 1.25 cups
- Active dry yeast – 1 tablespoon

The Instructions:

1. In your stand mixer bowl, combine the warm water, yeast, and half of the all-purpose flour to form a soft batter. Continue to add the remaining all-purpose flour until you get a soft dough that doesn't stick to the sides of the bowl. Continue to knead the dough with the hook attachment on low speed for four to five minutes. If you are kneading by hand, you will need to knead it for double the time.

1. Place the dough on a clean floured surface and separate it into six portions of equal size. Roll each portion into the shape of a ball. Cover all six of the dough balls with a clean kitchen towel and allow them to rise for fifteen minutes.

2. Using a rolling pin, roll each ball into a disk about .25 inch thick. Try to keep each disk of dough the same thickness all the way through so

that it cooks evenly. Allow the rolled out dough disks rise for thirty to forty minutes while covered with a clean kitchen towel. You know that they are ready when they are slightly puffy.

3. While the pita disks rise allow your oven to preheat to a Fahrenheit temperature of four-hundred and twenty-five degrees. Prepare a baking sheet by coating it with kitchen parchment.

4. Once the oven is done preheating and the pita disks have risen, transfer two of them onto the prepared baking sheet. Flip the pita disks over, so that the bottom side of the disk that had been resting on the counter is now facing upward. Spritz the dough disks with clean water.

5. Allow the pita disks to bake in the oven until they are lightly browned and have puffed up by several inches, about ten minutes. Sometimes, pita will refuse to puff up, and that's okay, too, you can use these as a flatbread.

6. Continue to bake the remaining pita dough after the first two are removed from the oven.

Italian Focaccia

This simple Italian Focaccia doesn't require kneading or the use of a stand mixer. You can easily make it with little hands-on work, allowing you to make a delicious and luxurious meal even if you have little time or energy to spare.

Chronic Kidney Disease Stage: 1-5/Dialysis

The Details:

The Number of Servings: 4

The Time Needed to Prepare: 15 minutes

The Time Required to Cook: 25 minutes

The Total Preparation/Cook Time: 40 minutes

Number of Calories In Individual Servings: 295

Protein Grams: 7

Phosphorus Milligrams: 74

Potassium Milligrams: 118

Sodium Milligrams: 59

Fat Grams: 7

Total Carbohydrates Grams: 49

Net Carbohydrates Grams: 48

The Ingredients:

- All-purpose flour – 2 cups
- Yeast – 1.25 teaspoons
- Warm water – 1 cup
- Olive oil – 2 tablespoons
- Italian herb seasoning – 1 teaspoon
- Garlic, minced – 3 cloves

The Instructions:

1. In a large bowl, combine the all-purpose flour and yeast, stirring well to incorporate the yeast evenly. Add in the warm water and continue to stir the mixture until the water and flour are completely combined. Cover the bowl with plastic wrap and allow the dough to chill in the refrigerator for at least eight hours, but up to twenty-four hours.

1. Grease a nine-inch round baking pan and then line it with kitchen parchment. Pour one tablespoon of your olive oil into the center of the lined pan. Add the dough into the pan, turning it over and coating it with the oil from the pan. Form a dough ball and then wrap the pan with plastic wrap, allowing it to rise in a warm location for two hours.

2. Preheat your oven to a Fahrenheit temperature of four-hundred and fifty degrees.

3. Drizzle the remaining tablespoon of olive oil over the dough ball, and then use your fingers to press the dough straight down into the pan. As you do this, you should create dimples in the dough with your fingertips. If the dough isn't quite reaching the edges of the pan, use your hands to stretch it.

4. Sprinkle the Italian seasoning and garlic over the top of the focaccia, and then place the pan in the center of your oven, allowing it to cook until golden, about twenty-five minutes. Remove the pans from the oven, and then use a spatula to remove the bread from the pan, transferring it to a wire cooling rack.

Cinnamon Swirl Loaf

This cinnamon swirl loaf is perfect on its own, but even better when it is used to make fresh toast in the mornings. You will love the fresh cinnamon flavor and find yourself making this delicious bread quite regularly.

Chronic Kidney Disease Stage: 1-5/Dialysis

The Details:

The Number of Servings: 4

The Time Needed to Prepare: 30 minutes

The Time Required to Cook: 30 minutes

The Total Preparation/Cook Time: 60 minutes

Number of Calories In Individual Servings: 326

Protein Grams: 7

Phosphorus Milligrams: 77

Potassium Milligrams: 87

Sodium Milligrams: 3

Fat Grams: 10

Total Carbohydrates Grams: 49

Net Carbohydrates Grams: 46

The Ingredients:

- All-purpose flour – 2 cups
- Water, warm - .75 cup
- Active dry yeast – 1.25 teaspoons
- Olive oil, light tasting – 3 tablespoons
- Cinnamon, ground – 1 tablespoon
- Truvia sweetener – 4 tablespoons

The Instructions:

1. Combine the warm water and active dry yeast together in a large bowl, whisking them until the yeast is dissolved. Allow this mixture to rest for five to ten minutes until the yeast is foam-like and bubbly.

1. Once the yeast has poofed, add in half of the Truvia, half of the olive oil, and the flour. Using the dough, hook on your stand mixer and combine this for three minutes. You will know that the dough is ready when it is soft yet pulls away from the sides of the bowl without sticking. If needed, you can add extra flour until it reaches this consistency.

2. Continue to knead the dough in the stand mixer until it is smooth and elastic, about seven minutes. Be careful to not over-knead the dough or it will turn tough.

3. Cover the bowl with plastic wrap and allow the dough to rise in a warm location until it has doubled in size, about thirty minutes.

4. Preheat your oven to a Fahrenheit temperature of three-hundred and fifty degrees and lightly grease a nine-by-five inch loaf pan. In a small bowl, combine the remaining half of the Truvia and the cinnamon.

5. Punch down the dough and then roll it into a rectangle nine inches long. Brush the dough with the remaining olive oil and then sprinkle the Truvia and cinnamon mixture over the dough.

6. Starting at the short side of the dough, begin to roll it into a tight log resembling cinnamon rolls.

7. Transfer the prepared cinnamon dough to the loaf pan, cover it with plastic wrap, and allow it to rise in a warm location for thirty minutes.

8. Place the risen dough in the preheated oven and allow it to bake until the dough is light and sounds hollow when tapped on about forty minutes. Remove the bread from the oven, let it rest for ten minutes, and then remove it from the pan, allowing it to cool on a wire cooling rack. Cool the bread completely before cutting it.

French Bread

Chronic Kidney Disease Stage: 1-5/Dialysis

The Details:

The Number of Servings: 6

The Time Needed to Prepare: 30 minutes

The Time Required to Cook: 30 minutes

The Total Preparation/Cook Time: 60 minutes

Number of Calories In Individual Servings: 330

Protein Grams: 8

Phosphorus Milligrams: 86

Potassium Milligrams: 98

Sodium Milligrams: 8

Fat Grams: 7

Total Carbohydrates Grams: 56

Net Carbohydrates Grams: 54

The Ingredients:

- All-purpose flour – 3.25 cups
- Warm water – .25 cup
- Hot water – 1 cup

- Active dry yeast – 1 tablespoon
- Honey – 1.5 tablespoons
- Olive oil – 3 tablespoons
- Egg white – 1 tablespoon

The Instructions:

1. In a large measuring cup, whisk the yeast and warm water together until it is dissolved. Be sure that the measuring cup isn't too small or else the liquid might expand too much and overflow. Allow the yeast to poof in the water for ten minutes, until it has expanded and become foam-like.

1. In a large bowl, mix together the hot water with the honey, olive oil, and half of the flour. Add in the yeast water that is done proofing. Slowly add in the remaining flour and continue to stir until the dough pulls away from the edges of the bowl. Allow the dough to sit for ten minutes.

2. On a floured surface, roll the dough into a long rectangle rolled up like a jelly roll and shaped like a French bread loaf. Smooth out the edges of the dough. Transfer the loaf onto a prepared greased

baking sheet and use a knife to cut four diagonal on the bread.

3. Using a pastry brush, coat the loaf with the egg white, which will give it a nice golden color during the baking process.

4. Allow the bread loaf to sit in a warm location, not covered, for forty minutes until it has risen quite a bit. Then, place it in a preheated oven set to Fahrenheit three-hundred and seventy-five degrees until it is golden, cooked through, and sounds hollow when you knock on it, about twenty to twenty-five minutes.

5. Remove the bread from the oven and allow it to cool completely before slicing.

Chapter 9: Desserts

While desserts should always be enjoyed in moderation, the desserts in this chapter have been created to be ideal for the kidney disease diet. While most desserts are full of sugar, these use natural alternative sweeteners that won't negatively affect blood sugar, and it keeps saturated fats from butter to a minimum. This means that if your chronic kidney disease is caused by diabetes or high blood pressure, you can still enjoy these desserts.

Cinnamon Apple Crisp

This apple crisp is perfect for autumn or any other day of the year. You will absolutely love how easy it is to assemble and bake, allowing you to have an inexpensive and delicious dessert in only a few minutes.

Chronic Kidney Disease Stage: 1-5/Dialysis

The Details:

The Number of Servings: 2

The Time Needed to Prepare: 10 minutes

The Time Required to Cook: 25 minutes

The Total Preparation/Cook Time: 35 minutes

Number of Calories In Individual Servings: 496

Protein Grams: 9

Phosphorus Milligrams: 180

Potassium Milligrams: 269

Sodium Milligrams: 5

Fat Grams: 18

Total Carbohydrates Grams: 77

Net Carbohydrates Grams: 71

The Ingredients:

- Apples, peeled and sliced – 2 cups
- Lemon juice – 1 teaspoon
- Truvia sweetener - .25 cup
- Cinnamon - .5 teaspoon
- All-purpose flour – 1 cup, plus 2 tablespoons
- Rolled oats - .25 cup
- Brown sugar Truvia sweetener - .3 tablespoons
- Butter, cold, cut into pieces – 3 tablespoons

The Instructions:

1. Preheat your oven to a Fahrenheit temperature of three-hundred and fifty degrees Fahrenheit.

1. Lay out your sliced apples in a loaf pan and then toss them with the lemon juice, cinnamon, and the regular Truvia sweetener.

2. In a small bowl, combine the flour and cold butter with either a pastry cutter or a fork until it creates a crumbly mixture. Add in the brown sugar Truvia and the oatmeal, and then sprinkle this crumble mixture over the apple slices.

3. Place the loaf pan in the oven and bake the crisp for twenty-five to thirty minutes, until the apples are tender and the topping is golden brown. Enjoy the crisp while it is still warm.

Vanilla Chia Seed Pudding

This pudding is quick and easy, but extremely delicious! Not only can it be made with strawberries, but other fruits as well! Customize this pudding to fit your taste or make it according to the recipe, either way, it is delicious.

Chronic Kidney Disease Stage: 1-5/Dialysis

The Details:

The Number of Servings: 2

The Time Needed to Prepare: 5 minutes

The Time Required to Cook: 0 minutes

The Total Preparation/Cook Time: 5 minutes

Number of Calories In Individual Servings: 106

Protein Grams: 3

Phosphorus Milligrams: 143

Potassium Milligrams: 135

Sodium Milligrams: 66

Fat Grams: 5

Total Carbohydrates Grams: 7

Net Carbohydrates Grams: 2

The Ingredients:

- Almond milk, vanilla, unsweetened - .75 cup
- Chia seeds – 4 tablespoons
- Vanilla extract – 2 teaspoons
- Truvia sweetener – 1 tablespoon
- Frozen strawberries, thawed – 3 ounces

The Instructions:

1. In a small jar, combine the chia seeds, unsweetened vanilla almond milk, vanilla extract, and Truvia sweetener. Ensure that the mixture is well combined so that the chia seeds don't form clumps. Allow this mixture to chill in the refrigerator for four to eight hours before enjoying. You might need to stir the mixture occasionally as it chills to ensure the chia seeds don't begin to stick together.
1. In a blender, puree the thawed strawberries, and then pour this puree over the chilled and set chia pudding. Enjoy the pudding immediately or store it in the fridge for up to four days.

Raspberry Frozen Yogurt

Whenever you are craving ice cream, all you have to do is reach for your blender to enjoy this raspberry frozen yogurt. Enjoy it either alone or with the addition of a little chocolate.

Chronic Kidney Disease Stage: 1-5/Dialysis

The Details:

The Number of Servings: 2

The Time Needed to Prepare: 5 minutes

The Time Required to Cook: 0 minutes

The Total Preparation/Cook Time: 5 minutes

Number of Calories In Individual Servings: 139

Protein Grams: 8

Phosphorus Milligrams: 123

Potassium Milligrams: 260

Sodium Milligrams: 27

Fat Grams: 0

Total Carbohydrates Grams: 27

Net Carbohydrates Grams: 22

The Ingredients:

- Raspberries, frozen – 6 ounces
- Greek yogurt, plain – .5 cup
- Lemon juice – 3 tablespoons
- Honey – 1.5 tablespoons
- Lemon zest – 1 teaspoon

The Instructions:

1. In a blender, combine the frozen raspberries, Greek yogurt, lemon juice, and honey until it forms a smooth and even consistency.
1. Either enjoy the frozen yogurt immediately for a soft-serve texture or place it in the freezer for one to two hours for a more solid consistency.

Skinny Cheesecake

This cheesecake is made much healthier by using a base of low-fat cream cheese and Greek yogurt, which is combined with Truvia as a sugar-free sweetener. This cheesecake is incredibly easy to make, and even someone new to the kitchen can follow this simple recipe.

Chronic Kidney Disease Stage: 1-5/Dialysis

The Details:

The Number of Servings: 6

The Time Needed to Prepare: 10 minutes

The Time Required to Cook: 60 minutes

The Total Preparation/Cook Time: 70 minutes

Number of Calories In Individual Servings: 199

Protein Grams: 8

Phosphorus Milligrams: 135

Potassium Milligrams: 182

Sodium Milligrams: 195

Fat Grams: 13

Total Carbohydrates Grams: 10

Net Carbohydrates Grams: 10

The Ingredients:

- Cream cheese, low-fat, at room temperature – 8 ounces
- Greek yogurt, fat-free – 1 cup
- Egg – 1
- Truvia sweetener - .33 cup
- Vanilla extract – 1 teaspoon
- Graham crackers – 1.5 ounces
- Olive oil, light tasting – 3 tablespoons

The Instructions:

1. Preheat your oven to a Fahrenheit temperature of three-hundred and fifty degrees and grease a five-inch round baking pan.

1. Place your graham crackers into a food processor and pulse them until they reach a uniform and fine crumb. Add in the light olive oil and pulse again until the fat is combined into the crumbs. Pour the crumb mixture into the prepared baking pan and firmly press down the cookie crumbs into the pan to form a crust. Set the pan aside while you make the cheesecake filling.

2. Clean the food processor, and then pulse together the Greek yogurt, cream cheese, Truvia, and vanilla extract. Process this mixture until it is fully combined, about one minute.

3. Add the egg into the food processor and pulse for a few seconds more to fully incorporate it into the cream cheese and yogurt base. Be careful not to over mix the cheesecake, as that will cause the top to crack during the cooking process.

4. Pour the cheesecake batter into the prepared graham cracker crust and allow it to cook in the preheated oven for thirty minutes. After the thirty minutes is up turn the oven off, leave the oven door closed, and allow the cheesecake to sit in the hot oven that has been turned off for thirty additional minutes.

5. After the thirty minutes of sitting in the oven that is turned off, remove the cheesecake from the oven, and allow it to sit on the kitchen counter until it reaches room temperature, at least four hours. Once room temperature, cover the cheesecake with plastic wrap and allow it to chill in the refrigerator for eight hours before slicing and serving.

Lemon and Honey Oatmeal Cookies

These cookies taste fresh and bright from the honey and lemon, but with a wonderful depth from the oatmeal. You can either buy oat flour pre-made at the store, or you can make your own by simply running some oats through the food processor. Either way, you will find that these cookies are incredibly simple and quick to make.

Chronic Kidney Disease Stage: 1-5/Dialysis

The Details:

The Number of Servings: 3

The Time Needed to Prepare: 5 minutes

The Time Required to Cook: 12 minutes

The Total Preparation/Cook Time: 17 minutes

Number of Calories In Individual Servings: 262

Protein Grams: 7

Phosphorus Milligrams: 297

Potassium Milligrams: 311

Sodium Milligrams: 15

Fat Grams: 8

Total Carbohydrates Grams: 41

Net Carbohydrates Grams: 38

The Ingredients:

- Quick oats - .5 cup
- Oat flour – 6 tablespoons
- Baking powder, low sodium - .75 teaspoon
- Coconut oil – 1 tablespoon
- Honey – 2.5 tablespoons
- Vanilla extract – 1 teaspoon
- Lemon juice – 1 teaspoon
- Lemon zest - .25 teaspoon
- Liquid egg – 1.5 tablespoons

The Instructions:

1. In a medium bowl, combine the quick oats, low-sodium baking powder, and the oat flour.
1. In another bowl, whisk together the liquid egg, honey, coconut oil, lemon zest, vanilla extract, and lemon juice.
2. Add the wet ingredients to the dry and combine the two until they are fully incorporated. Cover the

bowl with plastic wrap or a lid and allow it to chill in the refrigerator for thirty minutes.

3. Preheat your oven to a Fahrenheit temperature of three-hundred and twenty-five degrees and line a baking sheet with kitchen parchment.

4. Using a spoon, create six evenly-sized mounds of dough on the prepared baking sheet, each round of dough being one to two inches apart so that the cookies don't meld into each other. Use a fork and flatten the dough out into disks.

5. Bake the cookies in your preheated oven for twelve minutes, until they are set and starting to turn golden. Be careful to not overcook them. Remove the pan from the oven and carefully transfer the cookies to a wire rack to cool. Enjoy while warm or store them for later.

Carrot Cake Cookies

These carrot cake cookies are free of oils and granulated sugar, instead of using a small amount of honey and unsweetened apple sauce. Whether you are wanting these as a special dessert or a snack to take on-the-go, any fan of carrot cake will love these cookies!

Chronic Kidney Disease Stage: 1-5/Dialysis

The Details:

The Number of Servings: 3

The Time Needed to Prepare: 5 minutes

The Time Required to Cook: 12 minutes

The Total Preparation/Cook Time: 17 minutes

Number of Calories In Individual Servings: 179

Protein Grams: 5

Phosphorus Milligrams: 159

Potassium Milligrams: 187

Sodium Milligrams: 9

Fat Grams: 5

Total Carbohydrates Grams: 29

Net Carbohydrates Grams: 26

The Ingredients:

- Carrot, peeled and sliced – 1
- Honey – 3 tablespoons
- Apple sauce, unsweetened - .5 cup
- Rolled oats – 1 cup
- Walnuts, chopped - .25 cup
- Cinnamon, ground .5 teaspoon
- Ginger, ground - .5 teaspoon
- Nutmeg, ground - .25 teaspoon

The Instructions:

1. Preheat your oven to a Fahrenheit temperature of three-hundred and seventy-five degrees and line a baking sheet with kitchen parchment.
1. In a food processor, blend the carrots until they form a fine meal. Add in the honey, apple sauce, rolled oats, walnuts, cinnamon, ginger, and nutmeg. With the food processor, do five quick pulses, being careful to avoid over blending the mixture. Remove the blade from the food processor and use a spatula to finish combining the mixture.

2. Use a spoon or a small cookie scoop to make your cookie dough balls, each one containing two tablespoons of cookie dough. Use your hands to form the dough into two-inch disks and place these disks a couple of inches apart on the prepared baking sheet.

3. Place your baking sheet in the oven and allow the cookies to cook until they form a deep golden color around the edges, about twenty-five to thirty minutes.

4. Remove the pan from the oven and allow them to cool for five minutes before transferring the cookies to a wire cooling rack to complete the cooling process.

****

Download the Audio Book Version of This Book for FREE.

Copy, and Paste (text precisely) the link into your web browser to get started! https://tinyurl.com/wcobds6 or send an e-mail to: renaldietcookbook@gmail.com

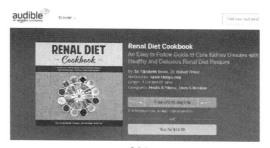

Conclusion

You likely had little knowledge about your kidneys before. You probably didn't know how you could take steps to improve your kidney health and decrease the risk of developing kidney failure. However, through reading this book, you now understand the power of the human kidney, as well as the prognosis of chronic kidney disease. While over thirty-million Americans are being affected by kidney disease, you can now take steps to be one of the people who is actively working to promote your kidney health.

With the help of Dr. Robert Porter and Dr. Elizabeth Torres, you now have all the information you need to succeed. You understand your kidney health better, you have learned of some of the new therapies now available and in the research stages, and you have been given over sixty recipes that can help you attain success and better health. Not only can these recipes help you improve your kidney functioning, decrease the risk of kidney disease, decrease mortality risk, and treat common conditions that coincide with kidney disease, but these recipes also taste amazing and can be incorporated into any healthy lifestyle.

If you found the knowledge and information imparted by Dr. Porter and the delicious and nutritious recipes shared by Dr. Torres helpful, then you should check out their other book. Their book, **Kidney Disease Diet,** will give you even more information on the biological function of kidneys, how chronic kidney disease and other kidney diseases affect your health, the prognosis of chronic kidney disease, and how you can take further steps, both with your diet and lifestyle, to better your health.

Thank you for reading the *Renal Diet Cookbook*. We hope that with the information you have learned, you will soon gain a healthier and happier lifestyle. You can enjoy gaining healthier kidneys, lower blood pressure, reduced cholesterol, and healthier blood sugar. By combining this book and a doctor's consultation, you can live better and longer.

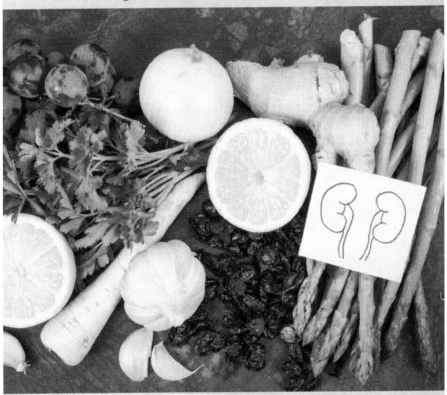

Printed in Great Britain
by Amazon